Cleanse and Detoxify Your Body

28 days to better health
using nutrient-dense whole foods

*You have tremendous power over your health, happiness and life . . .
it starts with what you put in your mouth.*

MW00947472

Name: Kellie Hill, NTP
ISBN-13: 978-1491259955
ISBN-10: 1491259957

dedication

to Mason

Best in
Health!

[signature]
11-18

Acknowledgments

Thank you to all my friends, family, clients, and various health care practitioners who have helped me along this journey. Each of you has offered support, wisdom, questions, and insight to healing from the inside out.

Special thanks to Scott Armstrong, Cynthia Becker-White, Teresa Bresnan, Karen Brooks, Tisa Cawthon, Dan & Jodi Chapman, Loren Fogelman, Dr. Brian Gross, my husband Doug Hill, my in-laws Lyle & Brenda Hill, Jim Jordan, Medford Food Co-op, Dr. Robin Miller, Christy Morrell, Paradux Media Group, Dr. Gary Reid, Debbie Richter, my mother Delores Rider, Nicole Sacks, Rebecca Schuh, Kirsten Shockey, Dr. Dan Smith, Dr. Jeff Taylor, and Jayson & Tina Tonkin. You have each provided wonderful guidance.

TABLE OF CONTENTS

The Body's Natural Detoxification System

Our bodies have a natural and automatic detoxification system. The body's defenses are made up of the liver, kidneys, colon, as well as healthy skin and immune system functions. This is necessary because our cells are constantly forming toxins as normal waste products of metabolism and, at the same time, we are exposed to toxic compounds in our food and environment.

Our toxin burden is created by multiple areas: cells release toxins into the blood, we ingest toxins, breathe them in, or absorb them through our skin. While in the bloodstream, antioxidants attach to the toxins neutralizing the toxins oxidizing capacity. With just a few heartbeats, the toxins are swept into the liver. A liver cell removes the toxin and this begins the detoxification processing which has two phases.

In phase 1, chemical reactions within the liver neutralize and may eliminate the toxin by one of three routes:
> 1. *Sending it into the bile to be eliminated in feces.*
> 2. *Sending it to the kidneys and into the urine to be eliminated.*
> 3. *Converting it into an intermediate compound, which will begin phase two.*

In phase 2, additional chemical reactions in the liver neutralize the intermediate compound and make it water soluble. At the completion of the process, the neutralized toxin can be eliminated.

This system works very well when not overloaded or receiving unidentifiable toxins. Our inherent detoxification system is designed to handle a natural diet packed with fresh, raw, alkalizing plant foods, heated plant foods, cultured vegetables, as well as high quality animal products. If we ate a natural diet, we would have all the antioxidants we need to protect our bodies from the oxidative damage caused by circulating toxins. We'd also have an abundance of all the nutrients the liver needs to perform both detoxification phases efficiently.

Unfortunately, we are inundated with toxic compounds daily in our foods, water, air, chemicals, as well as our own metabolic processes. This puts an extreme burden on our natural detoxification system. In foods alone, we are eating highly processed, unnatural foods the body has a difficult time identifying. These foods may be neutralized but instead of being eliminated they may be stored in fat tissues as part of the body's protection mechanism.

It is beneficial to help the body's natural detoxification system by removing major potential toxins.

Why Do We Need to Cleanse?

Today's society exposes us to toxins on a daily basis. We eat chemicals in foods such as hormones, pesticides, artificial dyes, and antibiotic residues. Our body works hard to break down these foreign substances while trying to pull nutrients from the same foods. For our own well-being these toxic compounds must be broken down, processed, and excreted from the body. The efficiency with which we are able to accomplish this is different for each person.

PARTIAL LIST OF SOURCES OF TOXINS:

pharmaceutical drugs	preservatives
air borne allergens	processed foods
food borne allergens	artificial sweeteners
water pollution	food additives
air pollution	dyes
pesticides	pesticides
chemicals	herbicides
caffeine	artificial flavoring
smoke	waste byproducts of normal metabolic function: ammonia, carbon dioxide, free radicals
cosmetics	
heavy metals	
cleaning products	

As you can see, we are being inundated with toxic compounds. Our body is designed to handle toxins and remove them naturally, but it can become overburdened with the amount of exposure in today's world and our detoxification system struggles to keep up. Eventually, these toxins can build up and cause disease. Cleansing gives your system a break.

"Everyone has a doctor in him or her;
we just have to help it in its work.
The natural healing force within each of
us is the greatest force in getting well.
Our food should be our medicine.
Our medicine should be our food."

~ Hippocrates

What Can a Cleansing and Detoxification Program Help With?

- Fatigue
- Lack of vitality
- Reduced mental clarity
- Food sensitivities
- Digestive and gastrointestinal problems
- Bloating
- Gas
- Constipation
- Diarrhea
- Forgetfulness
- Skin issues
- Racing heart

- Ulcers
- Leaky gut
- Learning issues
- Attention issues
- Sleeping difficulties
- Stuffy head
- Allergies
- Food cravings
- Forgetfulness
- Weight gain
- Dull hair
- Aches and pains

My Story

I doubt there is a cleanse or detoxification program out there that I haven't tried. There might be, but it's unlikely. Sometimes I tried them because I wanted to feel better. Sometimes I tried them to lose weight. Sometimes I tried them as an experiment. Some of them have value but I always ended up with issues afterwards. I started working on this program, for myself, many years ago. It's been changed for various clients again and again.

This program was put to the ultimate test last year. I had major surgery, was pumped full of lots of pharmaceuticals, and barely able to move for three months. I gained weight, felt horrible, and my body was having a difficult time getting the toxins out of my system.

I use many indicators to understand my toxic load from blood tests to hair analysis. One of the easiest, quickest, and cheapest ways I use is a live blood test. It is a test in which you can see with your own eyes the living condition of your cardiovascular health, immune system, toxic load, liver function, digestive function, hydration levels, and many nutrient deficiencies. It helps identify priorities to address to prevent future health problems and is an easy way to track progress on your nutrition and health program.

Working with a traditional medical doctor, naturopathic doctor, and the live blood analysis I learned that 60-70% of my blood was stacked up and congested with fibrin, an insoluable protein created as a response to bleeding and the major component of blood clots. I had a medium level of chemical and heavy metal toxins in my blood. I had a medium level of mycoplasma (parasitic bacteria), 5 protoplasts (markers indicating some level of leaky gut), very high levels of plaque, high levels of damaged white blood cells, and very high levels of dead fungus. There was a medium high level of oxidized proteins, which indicated my body was having difficulty detoxifying and repairing damage. In short, I needed to help my body cleanse and detoxify. Of course, I had just the right plan to follow.

The results speak for themselves. At my last testing I had an appropriate amount of fibrin; reduced inflammation in my blood; no indication of chemicals or heavy metal toxins; no indication of mycoplasma, only 1 protoplast; very little plaque; no damaged white blood cells; no dead fungus; very little oxidized proteins.

I couldn't be happier with the results. I feel better, look better, and think better. Yes, there's still a little more help I can give my body and I will, a couple times a year. If you're interested, join me for my yearly Spring Cleanse Group which includes a support system to help you through the Cleanse and Detoxify Your Body Program.

Why Whole Foods?

Nourishing yourself with nutrient-dense whole foods will provide the complex combination of vitamins, minerals, and antioxidants that are needed to cleanse the body and promote optimal health. This is real food, as close to its original form as possible, prepared to preserve or even enhance the nutritional value. Using whole foods allows us to remove the harmful foods and most common allergens while introducing more healing foods.

The foods chosen in this program will alkalize and purify the blood making it easier for the body to rid itself of wastes in a natural, authentic way. The body knows how to utilize whole foods and will absorb the largest amounts of high quality nutrients while giving the body's natural detoxification system a bit of a rest. Whole foods also allow us to "reset" our taste buds to healthy foods and away from artificial ones. Finally, whole foods, through the use of bone broth, will help repair any damage in the intestines.

Focus is placed on foods that support the liver which filters toxins, aids the body in metabolizing fat, protein, and carbohydrates, and transforms many toxins into harmless agents.

Focus is also placed on water and foods that support the kidneys which filter out waste and excess fluid from the blood, while regulating and releasing the right balance of sodium, potassium, and phosphorus for the body to function properly.

Processed foods are toxic and may have built up in your body. By using nutrient-dense whole foods you abandon all the "bad stuff". You lay the foundation for lasting change and optimal health.

Choosing organically grown foods can reduce the body's toxic burden. The more processing a food undergoes, the more toxins and the less energy and nutrient value it will hold. Where ever your budget will allow, try to choose local, organic ingredients. If you need to prioritize your organic purchases focus first on animal proteins, then bones for broth, oils, nuts, seeds, and vegetables. Health is more than just the absence of disease; it is the presence of vitality. Health is when you have the freedom to do anything you choose. Health is when you live in a way that creates both inner and outer peace. You can accomplish this by changing your food choices to nutrient-dense whole foods.

Food Types

To fully cleanse and detoxify the body we need a mix of heated, raw, and cultured foods as well as bone broth. Raw food is the primary cleanser and detoxifier. Raw food allows the body to not utilize our metabolic enzymes, which run our bodies. Cooked food is the primary nourishment. Cooked food supports cellular rebuilding after toxin removal. Cultured vegetables change and replenish the inner microbial balance. Cultured vegetables allow for profound changes in health as the ecology of the gut is improved. Bone broth will help repair damage to the intestines.

Most people understand raw and cooked foods, but cultured vegetables and bone both may be new.

Importance of Cultured Vegetables

The addition of cultured vegetables will increase bowel movements pulling toxins out of the body while replenishing and balancing the gut flora. Eighty percent or more of our immune system is located in the gut so balance is imperative for optimal health.

Look for cultured vegetables that have not been pasteurized, that are living foods with enzymes and natural probiotics. Find them in the refrigerated sections of health stores, on-line, or try the recipes included.

On-line resources include: www.immunitrition.com or www.wildmountainpaleo.com.

The key phrase to look for is **traditionally fermented or traditionally cultured**.

Though the term "fermented" sounds a bit distasteful, they are actually delicious. Fermentation is an ancient preparation and preservation technique, breaking down carbohydrates using microorganisms.

Importance of Bone Broth

Bone broth is used extensively in this cleanse because for centuries traditional households considered bone-broth a cure-all. In Asia, broth is traditionally consumed with every meal including breakfast. In traditional cultures in Africa, Europe, and the Middle East, broth is used to prepare the digestive system before eating. Broth, especially bone broth, was part of American culture for making stocks, soups, gravies, and stews until World War II.

Bone broth contains calcium, magnesium, potassium, phosphorus, silicon, sulphur, and other trace minerals in a form the body can easily absorb. Dietary sulfur is needed for sulfation, a pathway in Phase 2 detoxification. Sulfation is one of the weakest detoxification pathways for most people.

Bone broth contains gelatin which has an abundance of the amino acids arginine and glycine. Glycine is the most important for the neutralization of toxins. It is not an essential amino acid because the body can make it, if given the right building blocks, but the amount accumulated in the body is often depleted by a low-protein diet, stress, benzoates in soft drinks, and the use of aspirin. Gelatin is a colloidal substance, meaning it attracts digestive juices to itself. This allows for digestive action to be distributed evenly throughout the food so the digestive system can work less during cleansing and detoxification.

Finally, bone broth allows for less protein to be eaten which can ease digestive distress during the cleansing process without a loss of energy. Protein is a critical food source but during a cleansing and detoxification program it's important to allow the digestive system a rest while still providing maximum nourishment. For this reason the Cleanse and Detoxify Your Body Program uses bone broth as an ingredient for cooking as well as an option for a snack at any time.

Because bone broth is a staple in the program make sure you are purchasing only organic, grass-fed and pasture-raised bones. The same toxins you are trying to cleanse from your body may be stored in the animal and can be absorbed into your body. The cheapest choice is to check with your local butcher for bones or contact a local chapter leader at the Weston A. Price Foundation (http://www.westonaprice.org) for local options. You can get grass fed beef bones from US Wellness (http://www.grasslandbeef.com) which ships to all 50 states for free.

The combination of foods—raw, heated, cultured, and bone broth—is a nutritional powerhouse. You will have increased nutrient absorption, promote the growth of friendly intestinal bacteria, support immune function, and aid digestion.

My Experience:

When Lisa first came to see me her non-fasting glucose levels were extremely high, her A1C test (a common blood test used to identify and monitor diabetes) was extremely high, her blood pressure was high, and her cholesterol levels were high. After a longer preparation period, she eventually began the Cleanse and Detoxify Your Body Program.

Her non-fasting glucose levels are normal and have remained within normal range for almost a year. Her A1C test is within normal range and continues to lower within that range. Blood pressure has stabilized in the healthy range. Cholesterol levels continue to drop but are within the normal range.

Her doctors called to find out the secret to her success. It was easy to direct them to the Cleanse and Detoxify Your Body Program.

Why No Supplements?

There are many supplements that can support the body during detoxification and many people willing to sell them. The problem is that each person is an individual, with individual needs, individual efficiencies, and individual deficiencies. With private clients we may find an occasional benefit to using supplements. But, in the more generic form of a book, I feel it would be unethical, expensive, and potentially even dangerous to recommend various supplements that may or may not be helpful. My private clients have proven again and again that supplements are not required if you are using a nutrient-dense whole food diet for your cleanse.

If you would like to use supplements to support your detoxification, talk to your health care practitioner. He/she will be able to identify your best options and monitor your progress. Or, contact me for information regarding private client options. If you're interested, join me for my yearly Spring Cleanse Group which includes a support system to help you through the Cleanse and Detoxify Your Body Program.

This program has proven successful without supplementation.

My Experience:

After multiple surgeries, antibiotics, and pain killers, Susan wanted to detoxify her body. Her husband was willing to support her decision and they went on the Cleanse and Detoxify Your Body Program together. After the second week, I received the following email:

"Plan is working great, thanks. Haven't strayed once, am always full, love love love the recipes! I have even managed to lose about 2 pounds, and it's only day five [of elimination]. John is doing great as well and is sticking with me bite for bite. We both feel great with plenty of energy."

Ten days later she wrote:
"We made it! Finished day 22 today and we both feel terrific. I believe that we are whole foods converts. I never thought only food could make us feel so great. I don't even know if we want to try the eliminated foods we feel so wonderful."

Purification

What you drink is very important because it requires very little digestion and goes directly into your blood stream. Filtered water will help flush toxic compounds and is the recommended drink. If you don't like the taste of water try adding slices of lemon, cucumber, oranges, etc. to change the flavor. You'll be surprised; once your body begins to get fully hydrated you will actually crave water.

While cleansing, it is critical to stay fully hydrated. In order to figure how much water you should drink, take your current weight and divide by three. Two-thirds of your current weight is the number of ounces of water you should drink each day. Add more for exercising, warm or dry climates, and if you choose to sauna or steam (see *Other Cleansing Techniques*). For example: a 150 pound person needs to drink at least 100 ounces of water each day during the Cleanse and Detoxify Your Body Program.

When you drink liquids is just as important as which ones you choose. Your body can only metabolize about 4 ounces of water every 15 minutes, so downing 32 ounces all at once to get caught up on your goal is just going to make you visit the restroom frequently. Sip on water throughout the day. Try to refrain from drinking too much while eating to keep from diluting digestive juices.

Start with a big glass of water when you wake up. If you are having difficulty being hungry for breakfast, add 1-2 tablespoons of apple cider vinegar to the water first thing in the morning. This will get your digestive juices flowing. You can also drink a cup of water with 1-2 tablespoons apple cider vinegar about 30 minutes before lunch and dinner to help with digestion. Finish the day with a glass of water to help replenish what you will lose while you sleep.

Although staying hydrated is always critical, it is even more so during a cleansing and detoxification program. Approximately 62% of our body is made up of water. Healthy blood is between 85-90% water. Water is inside every cell and flows through the microscopic spaces between cells. Water is used to dissolve and carry away waste from our body. Without sufficient hydration the strain on the body can be damaging. During the Cleanse and Detoxify Your Body Program you are increasing the toxic burden in the blood in order for the toxins to become waste products and be removed. Increasing your water intake becomes critical to removing the toxins and purifying the blood.

Creating a Parasympathetic State

Your "state of mind" is important during the Cleanse and Detoxify Your Body Program. The more you can remain in a parasympathetic state the more success you will achieve. The parasympathetic nervous system is active during periods of digestion and rest. This system stimulates the production of digestive enzymes and stimulates the process of digestion and elimination. It reduces blood pressure, heart, and respiratory rates. While in a parasympathetic state you conserve energy through relaxation and rest.

To help bring about a parasympathetic state prepare your meals and sit down to eat. Start by taking 2-3 deep breaths with your eyes closed. Note the aroma. Open your eyes and take another 2-3 deep breaths while you really notice the visual appeal of your meal. Note the colors and textures. This will help relax and prepare your body to receive nourishment. Take your first bite, chewing until the food is almost a liquid. Note the taste, temperature, and texture. If you need help slowing down, put your utensils down between bites or eat with your non-dominant hand. Continue with each bite, really focusing on the food. Take a few deep breaths occasionally during the meal. Think of each meal as an experience to savor, not to be rushed or hurried.

My Experience:

"Working through the Cleanse and Detoxify Your Body Program provided self introspection on behaviors of mine that I had not considered before. I have read and been given advice in the past, that in a perfect world may have worked, but not in my hectic world of full time work, an active daughter, and family obligations. I needed something that was flexible and this program allowed me to achieve success at a pace that is attainable." Judy S.

A Note about Fasting and Juicing

When many people think of a cleansing and detoxifying program they think of fasting or raw juicing. Both of these techniques have merit. In fact, fasting is one of the oldest therapeutic treatments documented. And juicing has been successfully used for many chronic illnesses. Both fasting and juicing can be very healthful. In the Cleanse and Detoxify Your Body Program I've chosen not to recommend either technique for the following reasons.

First, fasting can feel like starvation, although it is not. People think if they don't eat for a day or two they will be starving and causing their body harm. They may be hungry, but they aren't starving. We live in a society with an abundance of food so we've become accustomed to eating whenever our stomach grumbles. But stomach grumbling only indicates that the stomach is empty, which is not the same as starving. Yet, I understand this concept is scary for many individuals. And, it's not necessary in order to participate in a healthy cleansing and detoxification of the body.

Most cultures and religions have successfully used fasting. If you would like to try a short term fast, 1-3 days, you can drink water and bone broth exclusively during this time. I recommend that you don't try this until you've completed the basic program as the fast will be more bearable because you will have already removed most foods with stimulating effects on the body. Fasting is an intense method of detoxification and can bring on a healing crisis (consult *Avoid A Healing Crisis*).

Second, juicing, similar to fasting can be very scary for people. Juicing can intensify the sugar content of drinks creating a stimulating effect on the body. One of the purposes of the Cleanse and Detoxify Your Body Program is to decrease sugar consumption. It is difficult to obtain enough protein and fiber with juicing so people frequently feel hungry. I have included a few smoothie recipes for those interested in drinking their meals, but I recommend chopping and blending the ingredients rather than juicing as the additional fiber will help with elimination and improve blood sugar regulation.

Avoid a Healing Crisis

Although the end result from a cleansing and detoxification program will feel amazing, the process can have some side effects due to the removal of toxic compounds. This is called a healing crisis. Our bodies are highly adaptive and your current toxic burden may even feel normal. During the program though you are disrupting this toxic state and you may feel the effects of the toxins being released into the bloodstream and digestive system before they leave the body. You may have an odd odor as the toxins leave through your largest organ, the skin. Your tongue may have a slight film when you awaken. In worse case scenarios you may feel lethargic or as if you are in the beginning stages of a sickness. This is unlikely since this program uses nutrient-dense whole foods rather than supplements, fasting, or juicing but the body will be trying to remove stored toxic compounds and you might notice the change.

You can minimize the risk of experiencing a healing crisis by:

- *Use Days 1-7 to prepare. Wean yourself off caffeine, alcohol, sugars, and processed foods.*

- *Stay fully hydrated. You can only flush toxins from the body by being properly hydrated.*

- *Eat beets at least once per day to support detoxification in the liver.*

- *Take time to get plenty of rest. Take the time to cleanse your mind while cleansing your body. Try meditating, deep breathing, or other relaxation techniques (read Other Cleansing Techniques).*

- *Do not over-exert yourself. Exercise facilitates the removal of toxins but a 30-45 minute moderate paced walk 4 times per week is sufficient.*

If you do begin to experience a healing crisis, consult the *Common Problems and Solutions* chapter and follow the instructions. If you do not feel relief within 48 hours, discontinue the program and consult your health care practitioner.

Common Problems and Solutions

CONSTIPATION
Cause: less food ingested. *Solution:* Increase water, add additional flaxseed to morning smoothies, increase vegetables.

CRAVINGS
See chapter Dealing with Cravings.

DIARRHEA
Cause: increased fiber intake. *Solution:* Usually will only last a few days but can be helped by Amaranth Porridge.

DIZZINESS
Cause: low blood sugar. *Solution:* Increase fluids and bone broth.

EXCESSIVE WEIGHT LOSS
Cause: less caloric intake in people with high metabolic rates. *Solution:* Increase calories, add flaxseed oil, nut, or fish oil to meals.

FATIGUE
Cause: low caloric intake. *Solution:* Increase amount of food, increase bone broth.

GAS
Cause: increased vegetable fiber consumption. *Solution:* Usually will only last a few days but can be helped by increasing water consumption.

HEADACHES
Cause: dehydration, caffeine withdrawal, liver congestion. *Solution:* Increase water consumption, increase beets. Try green tea or Teeccino.

HUNGER
Cause: low caloric intake. *Solution:* Increase amount of food, increase bone broth.

INSOMNIA
Cause: low blood sugar and liver congestion. *Solution:* Increase fluids and bone broth. Drink one cup bone broth before bed.

IRRITABILITY
Cause: low caloric intake. *Solution:* Increase amount of food, increase bone broth.

NAUSEA
Cause: bile stagnation. *Solution:* First thing in the morning drink lemon and water with a pinch of cayenne pepper.

Dealing with Cravings

One of the more difficult aspects of the Cleanse and Detoxify Your Body Program is that it is in an elimination diet. The meal plan includes no grains, no beans, no artificial fats, no dairy, no sweeteners, no caffeine, no alcohol, no tobacco, no stimulants, no refined sugars, no soy, no wheat, no eggs, and no corn. These are the major food allergens and intolerances for most people; removing them will help eliminate toxic compounds in the system. But, taking these out of your diet isn't always easy. Cravings will be decreased if you use days 1-7 to prepare; wean yourself off these foods.

If you do have cravings, here are some tools to help:

- *Change your environment if possible. Go for a walk, call for support from a friend or family member, play with a pet, anything to keep your mind off the moment.*
- *Drink a cup of water.*
- *Drink a cup of bone broth.*
- *Have a snack that's high in protein and good fat – nuts, seeds, avocado.*
- *Make a smoothie adding a tablespoon of coconut oil.*
- *Drink a cup of hot herbal tea. If necessary, add a bit of stevia.*
- *Floss, brush, and gargle with a natural mint or cinnamon mouthwash.*
- *Take a nap.*

My Experience:

Rose spent more than 30 years as a commercial painter and felt many of her health problems were related to the toxins she had worked around. She began the Cleanse and Detoxification Your Body Program.

"I am doing very well on the detox. I have lost 7 pounds. I feel good and usually full. I no longer crave yogurt and blueberries, wine, lattes, chocolate and most fruits. I have lost the craving for chocolate cake and most carbs. Your suggestions are excellent and varied and I usually find something that will satisfy me. Good job on this diet, Kellie."

At the completion of the program Rose said she had more energy than she had felt in years. "My complexion is clearer. My aches and pains are gone. I'm not stiff when I wake in the morning. I have a whole new spring in my step."

Who is this Program Safe for?

The Cleanse and Detoxify Your Body Program is safe for most people. As with any health program, specific results and reactions will vary with each person. If you have any hesitation about your ability to undergo a cleansing and detoxification program, get a physical exam by your health care practitioner. If you take regular medications, consult with your practitioner before beginning. Detoxification can change the rate of metabolism of certain medications and can clear them from your system faster.

Some people should not undergo this program without first consulting a practitioner:

- *Have a history of liver or immune disorders*
- *Children*
- *Nursing mothers*
- *Have a terminal or malignant illness*
- *Have a genetic disease*
- *Have an autoimmune disease*
- *Are chronically underweight*
- *Suffer from hyperthyroidism*
- *Have a mental illness*
- *Take any medications regularly*
- *Are pregnant*

My Experience:

Eden went to the hospital and learned she had a severe infection in her knee that spread throughout her body. Following emergency surgery she was given intravenous antibiotics for eight weeks. Suffering, she was then given pharmaceutical drugs to counter the antibiotic side effects. With minimal improvement, she went for another surgery three months later. After over six months of continual drug treatments, her body was ravished, depleted, and full of toxins.

She began the Cleanse and Detoxification Your Body Program. In the beginning, "the soups and smoothies seem to be the only foods I can tolerate well."

By the end, "All blood tests are fantastic. I have no symptoms of infection. Both doctors are very optimistic and amazed at the results. I'm not taking a single pill now but I continue to eat many of the Detox recipes."

FAQs

How often can I complete the Cleanse and Detoxify Your Body Program?

Most people enjoy completing the program 1-4 times per year. A shortened program may be helpful after medical illness, following indulgent holidays, when returning from traveling, or whenever you feel sluggish.

What outcomes can I expect?

Each person has a different experience. At minimum, most people learn to eat healthier and incorporate exercise. Frequently they have a new attitude toward food. Cravings will disappear. Others have less fatigue, more vitality, improved memory, reduced food sensitivities, improved digestion, less gas or bloating, better bowel movements, disappearance of skin issues, improved sleep, decreased allergy symptoms, less aches and pains, and weight loss.

What physical changes may happen?

Most notably there may be an increase in urination and bowel movements. This is a natural effect of the cleansing and detoxification of the body but shouldn't interfere with your daily activities. Although rare, people have experienced headaches, generalized aches, skin outbreaks, irritation, and fatigue – usually from caffeine or sugar withdrawal (solutions are provided in the chapter *Common Problems and Solutions*). These symptoms usually subside within three days. If you have any concerns, talk with your health care practitioner.

Isn't amaranth a grain?

No, it's technically a seed. It can be used to fulfill protein and calcium requirements. It contains more calcium and the supporting calcium cofactors (magnesium and silicon) than milk. It is unusually high in lysine, an amino acid that is low in most grains.

Why did you choose these vegetables?

These are extremely nutrient-dense and support detoxification.

I can't find grass fed bones.

Check with your local butcher for bones or contact a local chapter leader at the Weston A. Price Foundation (http://www.westonaprice.org) for local options. You can get grass fed beef bones from US Wellness (http://www.grasslandbeef.com) which ships to all 50 states for free.

What if I get really tired or lack energy?

If you are no longer experiencing withdrawal symptoms then your body may require a higher amount of protein while completing the program. Try the Seafood Breakfast and note if the feeling is lessened. If so, add an additional serving of fish to your breakfast meals.

Why is there so little protein?

The idea of the Cleanse and Detoxify Your Body Program is to remove digestive distress as much as possible while still absorbing the maximum about of nutrients. Proteins and fats spend the longest time in the digestive system, by minimizing them we allow the system more rest.

What types of fish can I use in the recipes?

Use any cold water, firm fatty fish that contains a good Omega-3 fatty acid profile such as salmon, mackerel, trout, tuna, halibut, cod, Pollock, haddock, etc.

Can I reheat already made bone broth?

Absolutely. Just don't reheat in the microwave because it denatures the amino acids in the bone broth.

Why do you insist on additional cleansing techniques?

A good cleanse and detoxification program is more than just removing toxins from your food. It's about cleansing your body, life, and space as a whole. Taking the time to focus on your health and prioritizing additional techniques will give you the ultimate success.

Do I really have to create positive affirmations?

Yes, don't skip this step. You have a lot of power over your health, happiness and life. It starts with what you put in your mouth, but what comes out of your mouth is just as important. Being in a positive mindset and having the intention for success helps creates your power.

The Program

The Cleanse and Detoxify Your Body Program is designed in three phases—preparation, elimination, and reintroduction. Read each section prior to starting the program. Familiarize yourself with the Other Cleansing Techniques chapter prior to starting.

During the elimination phase you will be drinking bone broth and following the recipes provided. Since this phase removes most of the common food allergens and reduces digestive distress there is ultimate choice in recipes so you can find foods that you will enjoy.

- *Plan your meals by choosing recipes for 3-7 days and shopping in advance.*
- *Choose a breakfast recipe, noting some can be made for more than one day at a time.*
- *Choose a lunch recipe, a cooked side dish, and a raw side dish for your mid-day meal; this is your primary meal each day.*
- *Choose a dinner recipe, noting some can be made for more than one day at a time.*

My Experience:

"I have grown to appreciate how medical science can be applied to help sustain life. It is this reason I searched for nutritional guidance. Kellie understands and applies the effects and functions of food in her program. Kellie uses her skills and knowledge to provide a program solely to enhance well-being. Kellie Hill's statement, "Everything you eat has a purpose and a plan... make it your purpose and THE RIGHT PLAN!" sums it up perfectly." Nichole L.

Days 1-7 Preparation

This is your transition week or weaning week. This week is to help ease you into the dietary changes. Choose a day to start and try not to begin when you have lots of parties, weddings, birthdays, etc. that may derail your program. For ultimate success, talk with your family and friends about your journey. Having their support will help you during the cleansing and detoxification process. Get your cabinets, crisper and appliances ready, read through the recipes, dust off your sneakers, sign up for daily affirmations on line, and locate a timer for your meditation or reflection times. It's time to get started!

During this week:

- *If you drink caffeine regularly, this is the week to start cutting down. If you can not completely remove caffeine prior to the next phase, substitute green tea or Teeccino.*
- *If you still smoke, schedule a visit to your practitioner to start a cessation program.*
- *Cut back to no more than two alcoholic drinks per week.*
- *Start increasing your water consumption.*
- *Make bone broth.*
- *Phase out dairy and gluten. Include no more than two or three servings of each over the course of the week.*
- *Eliminate processed sugar and refined carbohydrates. (See Dealing with Cravings.)*
- *Double your intake of greens – eat as many vegetables as you desire.*
- *Transition away from grains by cutting back to no more than ½ cup whole grain brown or wild rice once per day.*
- *Remove artificial fats and oils, such as margarine, hydrogenated oils, and partially hydrogenated oils.*
- *Remove any canola oil.*
- *If you haven't eaten beets in a while, make a beet recipe.*
- *Remove sweeteners including honey, agave, aspartame, white sugar, etc.*
- *Try a smoothie.*
- *Now's the time to experiment with some of the recipes*
- *Visit a health food store for available options.*
- *Visit a butcher to find grass-fed bones.*
- *Visit markets that sell organic foods. If you can afford organic, this can reduce the body's toxic burden. The more processing a food undergoes, the more toxins, less energy and nutrient value it will hold.*
- *Order any necessary items on line.*
- *Start completing your food journal.*

Completing Your Food Journal

Completing your food journal every day is very important. It will help you to:

- *stay on track*
- *remember which recipes were your favorites*
- *notice if any foods seem to cause digestive distress*
- *notice any mood changes*
- *remember to complete an additional cleansing technique*
- *remember to move or exercise daily*
- *enhance your well-being with daily positive affirmations*
- *identify potential allergens when reintroducing foods*
- ***see your results!***

Use the food journal to express yourself during the Cleanse and Detoxify Your Body Program. Write down everything you eat and drink, including all snacks, beverages, and water. If you notice any mood changes associated with a meal, snack, cleansing technique, or exercise, record it. If you notice any digestive changes associated with a meal, snack, cleansing technique, or exercise, record it. If you need help, read *Other Cleansing Techniques*. Write a positive affirmation every day and repeat it frequently. If you need help, see *Creating Positive Affirmations* chapter for suggestions.

My Experience:

"I've lost 33 pounds in the last five months. I have completely given up fast food. If we go out, we go to Mexican and I have meat and veggies. The whole family has picked up better eating habits along with the majority of my coworkers. It's amazing how when people see change they want to jump on the wagon. I am determined to become a success story. This time next year my goal is to be at least 80lbs lighter. I feel like a new person. Again, thank you!" Chandra L.

Days 8-22 Elimination Diet

Remember, the Cleanse and Detoxify Your Body Program is an elimination diet. It is designed to help decrease your toxic burden by focusing on foods that generally do not cause allergies or intolerances, are free of preservatives, pesticides, hormones, antibiotics, and other toxic elements.

During these weeks:

- **PLAN YOUR MEALS!** *Choose recipes for 3-7 days and shop in advance.*

- **PREPARE YOUR FOODS!** *Choose a breakfast recipe, noting some can be made for more than one day at a time. Choose a lunch recipe, a cooked side dish, and a raw side dish for your mid-day meal. Choose a dinner recipe, noting some can be made for more than one day at a time.*

- *Do not restrict calories.*

- *Try to eat so you are not hungry, but not over full. This is a cleansing and detoxification program, not a calorie restriction diet. Eat so that you are satisfied and if you are still hungry, eat additional vegetables.*

- *Eat at least three meals per day.*

- *Enjoy 2 Tablespoons of cultured vegetables with lunch (feel free to include more if you'd like).*

- *Drink bone broth for snacks and any time you desire additional food to avoid blood sugar crashes.*

- *Eat beets daily.*

- *Think about "eating with the sun". Breakfast is a light start. Lunch is your biggest meal of the day. Dinner begins the closing of your day.*

- *Drink warm water with lemon or apple cider vinegar 15-20 minutes before each meal.*

- *Avoid parties and social situations that do not support your cleanse.*

- *Meditate.*

- *Complete at least one additional cleansing technique.*

- *Drink plenty of water for purification*

- *Record meals and experiences in your journal.*

- *Write positive affirmations.*

- *Move to get the blood flowing: 35-40 minutes of walking at least 4 times per week plus 20-30 minutes of strength training 2-3 times per week*

- *Rest for at least eight hours at night – nap if necessary.*

- *Follow A Day At A Glance.*

A Day At A Glance

Each day during the elimination phase:

- *Meditate for 5 minutes upon rising*
- *Brush your tongue*
- *Utilize one beet recipe*
- *Eat breakfast in a parasympathetic state*
- *Drink bone broth if hungry*
- *In a parasympathetic state eat lunch with a cooked side dish, a raw side dish, and 2 Tablespoons of a cultured vegetables.*
- *Drink bone broth if hungry*
- *Eat dinner in a parasympathetic state – try to finish 3 hours prior to bed*
- *Drink bone broth if hungry*
- *Drink plenty of water for purification*
- *Record meals and experiences in your journal. Remember to write (and repeat) positive affirmations.*
- *Move to get the blood flowing: 35-40 minutes of walking at least 4 times per week plus 20-30 minutes of strength training 2-3 times per week*
- *Complete an additional cleansing technique*
- *Brush your tongue*
- *Rest for at least eight hours at night – nap if necessary*
- *Meditate for 5 minutes before bed*

Meal Planning

The difference between wanting to be successful and *being* successful is planning. It really only takes three steps.

FIRST, you *must* choose the recipes in advance. It's tough to come home from a long day at work, look in the fridge and try and figure out what to make with what you have. If your time is limited choose recipes with a larger number of servings so your foods are ready when you are.

SECOND, you *must* shop to have the correct ingredients available. It's *so* much easier to cook when you know you already have all the ingredients. Make a list of ingredients you'll need for the recipes. Double check the list at the end and cross off anything you already have. Organize your list to follow the flow of your grocery store. For example, write all the produce together, all the dry items, all the meats, bulk items, etc. There's no need to walk back and forth across the store to pick up forgotten items. Then shop.

THIRD, you *must* prepare the foods you will need *in advance*. Staying strong in the commitment you've made to yourself means being prepared. Since you already know what you're making, take a few minutes and do some prep work. For example, chop your onions for meals, vegetables for snacks or salads, and make your dressings, put single serve snacks in containers, etc

It only takes a little bit of time to ensure your success.

My Experience:

"I thought the hardest part of the program was going to be figuring out how to plan the meals. The transition week helped a lot in preparing. I had to stay on top of the plan but was surprised that it didn't take as much time as I thought. Now I plan each week out and we're never tempted to order out.

My blood tests continue to be great – cholesterol is down, blood pressure is down, thyroid is even, blood sugar is regulated. I continue to lose weight. It's been two months now [after the program] and I'm losing about 1lb every two weeks. My body seems to be much happier and well balanced. I feel so much better and have no pain. I have not taken any Aleve or pain relievers anymore." Kathy B.

Days 23-28
Reintroduction

The toughest part is over—Congratulations! I'm sure you feel fabulous and look great.

Many people are interested in adding some or all of the restricted foods back into their meal plans. You will be better able to determine if you have food sensitivities or allergies after the elimination part of the Cleanse and Detoxify Your Body Program. Only add one food every three days—so this part of the program may last more than a week depending on the number of foods you would like to reintroduce. It is important to pay attention to any symptoms you may be experiencing. If you notice bloating, gas, constipation, mood shifts, weight gain, etc. it's likely your body is not ready to assimilate the food. Allow your body to reset, by continuing the elimination diet and then try a different food. If you have no symptoms and feel good eating the food in question it's likely your body can metabolize the food and you can add it to your meal plan. Continue this pattern until you have tested all the foods you'd like to reintroduce.

You have treated your body gently and lovingly while providing it great nutrient-dense whole foods for the last three weeks. Honor yourself and take the reintroduction slowly, being aware of the toxins you choose to expose yourself to.

If healthy weight management was your goal, remember to watch portion sizes, include lots of vegetables, have healthy snacks available at all times, don't eat anything in excess, and keep a food journal.

My Experience:

"Through Kellie's wisdom, dedication, and guidance, I was able to stop taking numerous medications that my general practitioner had prescribed. He was astonished at the results produced by Kellie's program. I feel better, look better, I'm more active, and I'm sure I'm healthier. She is certainly an expert in determining what ails you and in figuring out a natural way to get your body to fix itself. Kellie doesn't just help you treat symptoms, she helps you fix yourself. This is what makes her special." Robert S

Other Cleansing Techniques

ACUPUNCTURE—Involves the insertion of very fine needles at precise points and then 30-40 minutes of relaxation. It can strengthen the body's natural detoxification organs, reduce cravings and withdrawal symptoms, while calming the mind. Find a certified practitioner at www.nccaom. org.

AFFIRMATIONS & ATTITUDE—Set your intentions for success. How we react to stress, our amount of play and laughter, and our ability to love and offer forgiveness all help to create a positive mental attitude. Remember to write down a few positive affirmations every day. It may be difficult to praise yourself but recognizing your strengths, your commitment, your resilience, and overcoming your insecurities is powerful.

BREATHE— Shallow breathing can create tense muscles, contributing to stress and fatigue while only using a small portion of our lung capacity. Any deep, mindful, and controlled breathing technique can have major benefits. Stop and focus on your breath. Breathe in deeply, expanding your chest as your lungs fill, hold the breath for a few seconds, and slowly release it.

DRY BRUSHING— Our skin is our biggest organ and one of the best ways to remove toxins. When the skin is clogged toxins can be reabsorbed into the body rather than eliminated. Purchase a natural bristle brush, use long, upward strokes starting at your feet and moving toward your heart. Brush your entire body toward your heart. This stimulates the lymphatic and immune system, which increases circulation while sloughing off dead skin cells. The best time to brush is right before you shower.

HYDROTHERAPY—Use hot and cold water to increase the flow of blood to various tissues. It creates circulation in organs that are under stress during detox. It is best to complete this technique on an empty stomach. In the shower, stand with water on your back, as hot as you can tolerate, for 5 minutes, then pure cold water for thirty fast breaths, repeat 5 minutes hot, cold again, one more cycle, dry off, and lay in bed under the covers for 30 minutes.

MASSAGE—Getting a massage may not specifically remove toxins but it can reduce heart rate, blood pressure and levels of stress hormones, enhance immune function, boost levels of endorphins and serotonin (the body's natural painkillers and mood regulators) and increase blood, while easing sore and achy muscles. Massage also removes the build up of lactic acid in muscles and promotes the clearing of normal byproducts of muscle metabolism.

OIL PULLING—Take one tablespoon of pure, organic coconut oil and swish it around in your mouth for 15-20 minutes. Move the oil around your mouth through sipping, sucking - pulling through your teeth. Spit out the oil, thoroughly rinsing your mouth out with water, and consume 2-3 glasses of water. Lipids in the oil help to extract toxins from the saliva. The absorbed toxins may create a thick, white liquid. The best time for oil pulling is when you wake up, before eating or brushing your teeth.

RELAX & REFLECT—As part of your self-care regimen take time to relax and reflect on your journey. It may be easy to commit to others, but make you a priority during this time. Schedule in relaxation – whatever that includes for you: read a book, watch a great movie, take a hike, sit in nature, soak in the tub, visualize, etc. At a minimum, get comfortable and try to relax for five minutes. Find a space just for you. Try to start and end your day feeling grateful for what you did accomplish.

SAUNA—Speeds up the metabolic rate and increases the body's ability to detoxify and eliminate harmful substances through the pores by sweating. Try 15 minutes followed by a cold water rinse, repeat up to one hour. Hydrate with one quart warm water before entering and sip throughout as well. If sauna is too difficult on your body, try a steam bath.

SUNFLOWER YOGA MOVE—Breathe in as you sweep arms up and breath out through mouth as you sweep arms down. Start with your feet apart and your toes turned out to the side at 45 degree angles. Inhale, reach the arms high, keep the shoulders relaxed. Exhaling, lower your arms to a "T" position while bending your knees and hinge forward at the waist. Remain neutral in the spinal column. Continue hinging forward and release the arms down so that they cross in a sweep near the ground. Shoulders may round at this part of the sequence. Inhale, begin sweeping the arms back up toward the starting position. Bring arms wide hitting the "T" position on the way up. Straighten the legs. Return to start position. Repeat 5-10 times.

SWEAT —Again, the organ we call skin eliminates waste and toxins, as much as a pound a day. By sweating you fully open the pores allowing the toxins to be pushed to the surface. Any type of sweating is helpful – exercise or sauna. Just be careful of overheating and/or dehydration. Without proper hydration you can overburden the kidneys and liver (see Purification chapter).

Creating Positive Affirmations

Affirmations make you conscious of your thoughts. It is important that your affirmations are positive. You are declaring your belief firmly and asserting it to be true. What you want to be true *is now* true.

Positive affirmations work because in order to make something happen, you have to decide what you want to happen. No matter what action you take, even in the briefest moment, you thought about it and decided you were going to take that action. Affirmations are the decisions you make to have something happen.

During the Cleanse and Detoxify Your Body Program you've already decided what you want to have happen with your body. The affirmations you use are simply you being in control of your thoughts. You are declaring to the universe what you want to be true.

With this program you're setting your intention to be healthier and less toxic. It's important to detoxify any negative thoughts and positively support your health, happiness, and goals.

Each day, focus on what success you want to have happen and repeat your affirmation to yourself – over and over and over.

Here are some suggestions to help you get started:

"Today's thoughts create my future. I am in charge."

"I love and approve of myself."

"I am eating foods that energize and nourish my mind and body."

"I have a lot of power over my health, happiness and life."

"I am beautiful and smart."

"Each step is a victory. I am improving now."

"I compare myself only to my highest self."

"The healthier I eat the better I feel in my mind and body."

"I am a light to this world."

"I let go of my fears, worries that drain my energy for no good return."

"I follow my dreams no matter what."

"My good health is increasing even more today."

"I have deep inner peace with myself as I am."

"Today is the first day of the rest of my life."

"I am the embodiment of success today! I am a champion!"

"I trust my inner light and intuition to guide me."

"Nervousness surrounding what I want to do is a good sign."

"I move forward, feeling self-confident every step of the way."

"I know the situation will work out for my highest good."

"I am happy in my own skin and in my own circumstances."

"I believe in my ability to unlock the way and set myself free".

"I am more than good enough and I get better every day."

"The past has no power and no hold over me anymore."

"I am deeply fulfilled with who I am."

The Recipes

Bone Broth

INGREDIENTS:

2 organic, pastured chicken carcasses or 1 full chicken or 3-4 lbs. bony chicken pieces

OR 7 lbs of organic, grass fed beef bones – 4 lbs bony bones + 3 lbs meaty bones

½ cup apple cider vinegar

2 bay leaves

1 Tbs peppercorns

2 onions, quartered

2 carrots, cut in large chunks

3 stalks celery, cut in large chunks

Filtered cold water

Herbamare or sea salt

Cracked pepper

DIRECTIONS:

1. If using beef bones, place all the meaty bones in a roasting pan and brown in the oven at 350 degrees until well-browed (30-60 minutes). You can skip this step if in a hurry.

2. Place all non-meaty marrow bones into a stockpot, add the vinegar and let sit while other bones are browning.

3. Add the bay leaves, peppercorns, and vegetables to the stockpot.

4. Add the browned bones to the stockpot. Deglaze the roasting pan with hot water and scrape up all the brown bits. Add this liquid to the stockpot.

5. Add additional filtered water to cover the bones and vegetables.

6. Bring to a boil. Remove the foam that rises to the top. Do not remove the floating fat. Reduce heat, cover and simmer at least 24 hours.

7. Scoop out amount desired to drink; season with herbamare, sea salt, and pepper if desired. Replenish with filtered water. You can leave the bone broth on the burner or in a slow cooker for up to a week.

8. After a week, remove the bones with a slotted spoon or tongs. Reduce the liquid until desired taste for stock. Strain the broth into a large container. Allow to cool in the refrigerator. You can remove the congealed fat if you'd like.

Cultured Vegetables

Sauerkraut

INGREDIENTS:

Head of cabbage (white or ½ white and ½ red)

2 carrots

1-2 Tbs sea salt

DIRECTIONS:

1. Thinly shred the cabbage. Grate carrots. Place in large bowl.

2. Add salt. Knead the mixture well until very juicy. Add a little water if not enough juice is formed.

3. Pack mixture into a glass or enameled bowl. Press firmly to remove all trapped air. Any air will rot the mixture instead of fermenting. Mixture should be drowned in its own juice.

4. Place a plate on top of the cabbage that is a bit smaller in diameter than the bowl. This will allow fermentation gases to escape. Place a heavy item on top of the plate to keep mixture constantly submerged in its own juices.

5. Cover with kitchen towel. Place in dark area for 5-7 days.

HELPFUL TIP: You can ferment the mixture in glass jars. Ensure mixture is fully submerged in its own juice. Leave at least an inch of space at the top of the jar to allow the mixture to expand during fermentation.

Fermented Vegetables #1

INGREDIENTS:

Whole cabbage

Medium size beet

1 tsp dill seeds or dill herb

5 garlic cloves

2 Tbs sea salt

Vegetable starter (optional)

Filtered water

DIRECTIONS:

1. Roughly chop cabbage. Peel and slice beet. Peel garlic.

2. Place all items in large enameled pan or glass jar. If vegetables fill less than half of container, add more. Add water until about 1 inch from top.

3. Place a small plate on top to keep the vegetables completely submerged in the brine.

4. Cover with a kitchen towel. Place in a dark area and allow to ferment for 1-2 weeks.

5. To stop the fermentation, place container in the refrigerator.

6. As the vegetables begin to get low, add fresh vegetables, some sea salt, top with water and ferment again at room temperature.

Fermented Vegetables #2

INGREDIENTS:

3 lbs sweet red peppers

1 medium sweet onion

1 lb jalapeno peppers

4 garlic cloves

2 tsp sea salt

Filtered water

DIRECTIONS:

1. Chop peppers, onions, and garlic in a food processor.

2. Place all items in large enameled pan or glass jar. If vegetables fill less than half of container, add more. Add water until about 1 inch from top.

3. Place a small plate on top to keep the vegetables completely submerged in the brine.

4. Cover with a kitchen towel. Place in a dark area and allow to ferment for 1-2 weeks.

5. A white scum will develop, this is normal.

6. To stop the fermentation, skip any scum from the top and place container in the refrigerator.

Breakfasts

Amaranth Porridge

INGREDIENTS:

½ cup amaranth

½ cup warm filtered water

1 Tbs fresh lemon juice

¼ tsp sea salt

½ cup milk alternative (almond milk, brown rice milk, cashew milk, coconut milk, hazelnut milk, hemp milk, oat milk—not soy)

½ Tbs fresh ground flaxseeds

DIRECTIONS:

1. Heat skillet over high heat. Add amaranth and toast, stirring constantly until fragrant. It will smell like popcorn.

2. Place amaranth in a small pot. Add water and lemon juice. Stir and cover. Allow to soak for at least overnight, but 24 hours is better.

3. Bring milk alternative to almost boiling. Add amaranth, reduce heat, cover and simmer 3-5 minutes.

4. Grind flaxseed.

5. Remove amaranth from heat, stir in flaxseed and let stand for a few minutes.

6. Serve. You can add additional milk alternatives, nuts, and/or coconut.

MAKE AHEAD ALERT: Amaranth must soak at least overnight, but 24 hours is better.

Serves 2

Breakfast Bake

INGREDIENTS:

1 ⅔ cup water

2 ½ Tbs fresh lemon juice

1 Tbs fresh ground flaxseed

3 Tbs very hot water

1 ¼ cup almond flour

Pinch fine sea salt

¼ tsp baking soda

1 tsp cinnamon

½ tsp allspice

⅛ tsp stevia

¼ cup coconut oil, melted

1 tsp vanilla

½ cup shredded coconut

½ cup pumpkin seeds

½ cup sunflower seeds

¼ cup chopped almonds

¼ cup cranberries

½ cup milk alternative
(almond milk, brown rice milk,
cashew milk, coconut milk,
hazelnut milk, hemp milk,
oat milk—not soy)

DIRECTIONS:

1. Mix water and lemon juice. Add seeds and almonds. Stir. Cover and leave in a warm place overnight.

2. Preheat oven to 350 degrees.

3. Mix ground flaxseed and hot water. Allow to sit to form a paste.

4. Mix almond flour, salt, soda, cinnamon, allspice, and stevia.

5. Mix melted coconut oil and vanilla.

6. Add wet ingredients and flaxseed mixture to dry ingredients. Mix well.

7. Add remaining ingredients and mix well.

8. Place in 8 x 8 pan. Using a piece of parchment paper press mixture into pan to flatten.

9. Bake for 25 minutes. Serve warm or cold with milk alternative.

MAKE AHEAD ALERT: Seeds and nuts must soak overnight.

INTERESTING TIDBIT: Some clients have found this recipe to make more of a breakfast bar (which is what I was originally trying for) while I've always ended up with chunks and crumbles. Either way is delicious!

Makes 6 servings

Cauliflower Pancakes

INGREDIENTS:

1 head cauliflower

2 Tbs BPA-free canned coconut milk

6 Tbs almond flour

2 Tbs coconut flour

1 tsp baking powder

¼ tsp nutmeg

2 tsp cinnamon

2 Tbs cashew butter

Coconut oil

½ cup organic, unsweetened applesauce or pumpkin purée

DIRECTIONS:

1. Chop cauliflower and steam for 10 minutes.

2. Place cauliflower in food processor. Add coconut milk. Process until smooth.

3. Mix together almond flour, coconut flour, baking powder, nutmeg, and cinnamon.

4. Mix together cauliflower, flour mixture, and cashew butter.

5. Heat griddle or skillet until a water drop "jumps".

6. Wipe griddle with a thin coating of coconut oil. Use 2 Tbs of pancake mix and flatten with a spatula. Cook for 4-5 minutes on each side.

7. Top with applesauce or pumpkin purée.

Makes 8 pancakes—serves 1-2

Cleansing Smoothie

INGREDIENTS:

½ large cucumber, peeled

2 stalk kale

2 romaine lettuce leaf

2 stalks celery

2 broccoli stems

½ + inch piece of ginger root, peeled

4-8 Tbs water

½ cup pineapple chunks (optional)

DIRECTIONS:

1. Place cucumber, kale, romaine, celery, broccoli, and ginger in blender, Vita-Mix, or juicer. If using a blender, chop ingredients finely.

2. Begin processing. Add water one tablespoon at a time if using a blender or Vita-Mix.

3. Process until smooth. Add additional ginger root to taste.

4. Add pineapple chunks for additional sweetness if needed.

5. Drink within 10 minutes.

Serves 1

Detox Smoothie

INGREDIENTS:

1 ½ cups aloe vera juice

⅓ cup fresh parsley

1 ¾" wedge of red cabbage

½ cup kale

1" piece of fresh ginger, peeled

½ lemon, include as much pith as possible

½ small beet or ¼ cup beet juice (depending on power of blender)

Pinch cayenne pepper

Stevia (optional)

1 cup ice cubes if desired

DIRECTIONS:

1. Chop ingredients finely if using a blender. Add ingredients to blender or Vita-Mix . Add water to desired consistency.

Serves 1

Hash

INGREDIENTS:

½ small sweet potato, cooked and cooled

1 tsp coconut oil

1 Tbs coconut aminos

½ Tbs bone broth

¼ cup onion, finely chopped

1 garlic clove, pressed

¼ cup pepper, chopped

⅛ tsp chili powder

⅛ tsp turmeric

⅛ tsp paprika

⅛ tsp dried rosemary or ¼ Tbs fresh rosemary

⅛ tsp dried basil or ¼ Tbs fresh basil

1 Tbs bacon crumbles (optional)

Sea salt

Fresh ground pepper

DIRECTIONS:

1. Cook sweet potato for 40-45 minutes at 350 degrees. Allow to cool.

2. Chop onion and press garlic. Allow to sit for 5-10 minutes. Chop pepper.

3. Mix coconut aminos and broth.

4. Sauté onion, pepper, dried herbs if using, in coconut oil for 2-3 minutes.

5. Add potato and sauté for 2-3 minutes or until warmed through.

6. Add garlic, and sauté for another minute.

7. If ingredients begin to stick during sautéing add ½ of aminos/broth sauce.

8. Add any remaining sauce, seasonings, and fresh herbs. Stir.

9. Top with bacon crumbles, if using. Salt and pepper to taste.

MAKE AHEAD ALERT: Cook sweet potato up to five days in advance and store in refrigerator.

Serves 1

Liver Detox Smoothie

INGREDIENTS:

½ small beet or ¼ cup beet juice

3 to 4 beet green leaves

3 to 4 dandelion leaves

¼ to ½ lemon

½-1 apple

1 inch fresh ginger

1 cup water

DIRECTIONS:

1. Chop ingredients finely if using a blender. You can blend the beet in your blender, if your blender has a powerful motor.

2. Add ingredients to blender. Blend to desired consistency.

Serves 1

Power Breakfast

INGREDIENTS:

⅓ 3 cup warm filtered water

½ Tbs fresh lemon juice

1 Tbs flaxseeds

2 Tbs sesame seeds

2 Tbs sunflower seeds

1 Tbs chia seeds

½ Tbs coconut flakes

¼ cup blueberries

milk alternative (almond milk, brown rice milk, cashew milk, coconut milk, hazelnut milk, hemp milk, oat milk—not soy)

DIRECTIONS:

1. Mix water and lemon juice. Add sesame seeds, and sunflower seeds. Stir. Cover and leave in a warm place overnight.

2. Add chia and flaxseeds and grind seed mixture together in coffee grinder.

3. Place seeds in cereal bowl.

4. Add warm milk if desired. Add milk or milk substitute. Stir if desired.

5. Top with chopped nuts and/or additional coconut flakes to desired taste.

6. Can be served hot or cold.

MAKE AHEAD ALERT: Sesame and sunflower seeds must soak overnight.

Serves 1

Scramble

INGREDIENTS:

¼ cup onions

1 clove garlic

¼ cup peppers

¼ cup broccoli

3 asparagus spears

¼ cup mushrooms

3 kalamata olives

1 Tbs coconut oil

½ cup cooked cubed chicken (optional)

2 Tbs chopped herbs (rosemary, oregano, cilantro, thyme, basil, or parsley)

½ tsp. paprika

¼ tsp. turmeric

DIRECTIONS:

1. Dice onions and mince garlic. Allow to sit for 5-10 minutes.

2. Chop peppers, broccoli, and asparagus. Slice mushrooms. Halve olives.

3. Heat skillet, add oil until melted. Add all ingredients except garlic, herbs, and seasonings. Sauté until vegetables are tender but still crisp.

4. Add garlic and sauté for another minute.

5. Top with herbs and seasonings. Serve.

Serves 1

Seaside Breakfast

INGREDIENTS:

½ tomato

½ avocado

4-6 shrimp (optional)

Salsa (optional)

Balsamic vinegar (optional)

Pinch of fresh herbs (rosemary, oregano, thyme, or basil)

Sea salt

Fresh ground white pepper

DIRECTIONS:

1. Slice tomato and avocado.

2. Grill tomato slices and shrimp. Or pan fry using a small coating of coconut oil.

3. Place tomato slices on plate. Top with avocado slices. Top with shrimp.

4. Drizzle salsa or balsamic vinegar on top, if using.

5. Add seasonings to taste.

Serves 1

Lunches

Baked Fish

INGREDIENTS:

1 lb fresh fish

2 cloves garlic

2 leeks

1 onion

1 ½ cups bone broth

1 tsp dried thyme

1 cup rice wine vinegar

1 ½ Tbs miso paste

½ tsp turmeric

1 head cauliflower

½ pound brussel sprouts

2 Tbs dried parsley

Pinch of cayenne pepper

Pinch of paprika

DIRECTIONS:

1. Preheat oven to 475 degrees.

2. Cut off green tops of leeks and remove tough outer leaves. Cut off root end of leeks. Cut in half lengthwise. Fan out and rinse well but keep whole. Cut into 2-inch lengths and then cut into thin strips or ribbons.

3. Press garlic, and slice onion. Allow leeks, garlic and onion to sit for 5-10 minutes.

4. Cut fish into four servings. Pat dry.

5. In a small bowl, combine broth, thyme, rice wine vinegar, miso paste, turmeric, and garlic.

6. Slice cauliflower. Half or quarter brussel sprouts.

7. Place vegetables in large baking dish.

8. Arrange fish on top. Pour mixture over fish. Sprinkle with parsley, cayenne, and paprika.

9. Bake for 15-20 minutes until fish flakes easily with fork and vegetables are tender crisp.

Serves 4

Blackened Fish

INGREDIENTS:

1 lb fresh fish
1 Tbs garlic powder
1 Tbs dried parsley
1 Tbs dried basil
2 tsp dried thyme
1-2 tsp cayenne pepper
1 tsp turmeric
1 tsp paprika
1 tsp sea salt
¼ tsp ground white pepper
1-2 Tbs coconut oil

DIRECTIONS:

1. Cut fish into four servings.

2. Mix seasonings together and place on flat plate.

3. Place fish in seasonings making sure to coat all sides.

4. Heat skillet over medium high heat. Add coconut oil to melt. Make sure oil is hot but not smoking.

5. Add fish and cook for about 3 minutes per side.

6. Serve.

Serves 4

Chicken and Bok Choy

INGREDIENTS:

1 bunch green onions

2 cloves garlic

2 Tbs coconut oil

2 Tbs fresh minced ginger

2 skinless, boneless organic chicken breasts, cut into bite-sized pieces

1½ cups sliced fresh shiitake mushrooms

4 cups chopped bok choy

2 Tbs coconut aminos

1 Tbs rice vinegar

salt and white pepper to taste

pinch of red pepper flakes

DIRECTIONS:

1. Chop green onions, press garlic and allow to sit for 5-10 minutes.

2. Heat oil in skillet. Add green onions and sauté for 2 minutes.

3. Add ginger and garlic. Sauté for another minute.

4. Add chicken and continue to sauté.

5. After 2-3 minutes, add shiitake mushrooms and bok choy. Continue to sauté for another 3-4 minutes, and then add coconut aminos, rice vinegar, salt, and pepper.

Serves 4

Cilantro Fish

INGREDIENTS:

1 lb fresh fish

Sea salt

Fresh ground white pepper

1 onion

2 cloves garlic

2 stalks celery

2 carrots

1 tsp fresh ginger, peeled and minced

1 Tbs coconut oil

1 ½ cup bone broth

½ cup fresh cilantro, chopped

DIRECTIONS:

1. Preheat oven to 375 degrees.

2. Chop onion and mince garlic. Allow to sit for 5-10 minutes.

3. Cut fish into four servings. Pat dry with paper towel. Sprinkle with sea salt and pepper.

4. Bake for 20 minutes or until fish flakes easily with a fork.

5. While fish is baking, chop celery, carrots, cilantro, and mince ginger.

6. Heat coconut oil in pan over medium heat. Sauté onions, celery, carrots, and ginger for about 10 minutes. Add garlic and sauté for an additional minute.

7. Add broth. Simmer, partially covered until the vegetables are tender, about 10 minutes.

8. Purée vegetables in a blender. Add cilantro and stir to mix.

9. Pour sauce over fish and cooked greens of choice.

Serves 4

Coconut Chicken

INGREDIENTS:

4 green onions

1 leek

½ medium onion

4 garlic cloves

1 pound organic, boneless, skinless chicken breasts

2 heads of broccoli

1 red pepper

2 tsp coconut oil

½ cup smooth almond butter

1 cup BPA-free canned coconut milk

2 Tbs fresh lemon juice

2 Tbs coconut aminos

1 Tbs fish sauce

½ cup warm water

¼ cup roasted nuts (optional)

¼ cup dried cranberries (optional)

DIRECTIONS:

1. Cut off green tops of leeks and remove tough outer leaves. Cut off root end of leeks. Cut in half lengthwise. Fan out and rinse well but keep whole. Cut into 2-inch lengths and then cut into thin strips or ribbons.

2. Chop white parts of green onion, chop regular onion, mince garlic and allow to sit for 5-10 minutes.

3. Cube chicken. Chop red pepper and broccoli, including stalks.

4. Sauté onions in coconut oil until softened. Add garlic and sauté for another 1-2 minutes until onions are slightly brown and garlic is fragrant.

5. In a blender, combine cooked garlic and onions with almond butter, coconut milk, lemon juice, coconut aminos, fish sauce and water. Blend until smooth.

6. In a large skillet, combine blended sauce, chicken cubes, broccoli, red pepper, and onion. Cover and cook until chicken is done, about 15 minutes.

7. Add optional roasted nuts and cranberries before serving.

8. Good warm or cold.

Serves 4

Foolproof Fish

INGREDIENTS:

4-4 oz wild caught fish fillets

2 tsp grated lemon zest

4 Tbs chopped fresh mixed herbs
(oregano, basil, parsley, rosemary, chives, tarragon)

Freshly ground white pepper to taste

2 Tbs white wine vinegar

2 Tbs white grape juice

4 Tbs macadamia nut oil

1 Tbs Dijon mustard

DIRECTIONS:

1. Preheat oven to 375°F

2. Rinse fish under cold water and pat dry with paper towel.

3. Arrange each fillet on a sheet of parchment paper.

4. Sprinkle with lemon zest, fresh herbs, and pepper.

5. Combine vinegar, juice, oil and mustard and pour over fish, making sure the edges of the paper are folded up to hold sauce.

6. Tightly seal the parchment paper to create a packet by double folding edges and sides.

7. Arrange on a baking sheet and bake about 15 minutes, until fish is tender and easily flakes with a fork.

Serves 4

Halibut—Quick & Easy

INGREDIENTS:

2 cloves garlic

1 lb fresh halibut

Juice of one lemon

Sea salt

Fresh ground pepper

2 Tbs coconut oil

2 sprigs fresh thyme

DIRECTIONS:

1. Preheat oven to 450°F

2. Press garlic cloves and allow to sit for 5-10 minutes.

3. Pat the halibut dry and cut into four pieces.

4. Rub a little lemon juice on halibut, sprinkle with sea salt and fresh ground pepper.

5. Heat coconut oil in large skillet until very hot but not smoking.

6. Sear halibut, about a minute on each side.

7. Add thyme and garlic cloves. Place skillet in oven until halibut is cooked through, about 4 minutes.

8. Add remaining lemon juice to pan and swirl to infuse flavors.

9. Drizzle pan dripping "sauce" over fish and greens of choice. If there isn't enough sauce left, add a little olive oil and swirl around pan.

Serves 4

Poached Fish

INGREDIENTS:

2 cloves garlic

¼ cup white wine vinegar

½ cup bone broth

¼ cup white grape juice

Juice of one lemon

Juice of one orange

1 lbs fish fillets

1 ½ tsp dried parsley

1 ½ tsp dried rosemary

Sea salt and white pepper to taste

DIRECTIONS:

1. Press garlic and allow to sit for 5-10 minutes.

2. Cut fish into four servings.

3. In a large skillet, heat vinegar, broth, and juices over medium heat, just until bubbling.

4. Slide fillets into the poaching liquid. Sprinkle with parsley, rosemary, garlic, salt, and pepper.

5. Bring back to a slow boil. Reduce heat to medium.

6. Poach until fish flakes easily with a fork, about 10 minutes.

Serves 4

Seared Ahi Tuna

INGREDIENTS:

1 pound fresh premium grade Ahi tuna

¼ cup paprika

¼ cup black sesame seeds

¼ cup white sesame seeds

2 Tbs garlic granules

1 tsp onion powder

1 tsp dried thyme

⅛ tsp stevia

1 tsp coarse sea salt

2 tsp cayenne pepper

1 tsp white pepper

1 tsp black pepper

DIRECTIONS:

1. Cut tuna into four servings. Pat dry with a paper towel.

2. Mix seasonings. Save approximately ½ of the seasoning mix for another meal.

3. Place seasoning mix on a flat plate. Place fish pieces individually on plate and lightly coat all sides. Shake off excess seasoning.

4. Heat skillet over medium to high heat. Add coconut oil and heat. Do not allow oil to smoke.

5. Sear the tuna on all four sides, lowering the heat if necessary to avoid burning the seasoning.

6. Place tuna on plates and allow to sit for another minute. Cut across the grain into ¼ inch slices.

COOKING TIP: If you prefer tuna more well done, use an ovenproof skillet and finish cooking in a 450 degree oven for 4-5 minutes. I recommend trying tuna seared first before choosing additional cooking.

Serves 4

Steamed Fish

INGREDIENTS:

1 lb fish

6 cloves garlic

Juice of one lemon

2 tsp miso paste

4-6 rosemary sprigs

4-6 thyme sprigs

Sea salt and white pepper to taste

DIRECTIONS:

1. Press garlic and allow to sit for 5-10 minutes.

2. Fill the bottom of a steamer or pot with 2 inches of water.

3. Cut fish into four servings.

4. Mix garlic, juice, and miso to make sauce. Remove leaves from rosemary and thyme sprigs.

5. When water is boiling, place fish in steamer basket. Pour sauce over fish. Top with rosemary and thyme leaves.

6. Steam for 7-10 minutes or until fish flakes easily with a fork.

Serves 4

Stir-Fried Chicken

INGREDIENTS:

1 onion, sliced

1 pound boneless, skinless organic chicken breast

1 cup fresh or frozen asparagus, chopped

1 cup kohlrabi orb, chopped

Kohlrabi leaves (from orbs), finely chopped

1 cup mushrooms, sliced

½ bunch dandelion greens, finely chopped

1 cup broccoli, chopped

1 cup cabbage, shredded

1 Tbs coconut oil

Bone broth, as needed

MARINADE:

6 cloves garlic, pressed

5 tsp coconut aminos

2 tsp arrowroot

1 inch slice fresh ginger, peeled and minced

6 sliced green onions

DIRECTIONS:

1. Press garlic, and slice onion. Allow to sit for 5-10 minutes.

2. Cut chicken breast into ½ inch cubes.

3. Whisk together marinade. Place chicken cubes in marinade.

4. Chop remaining vegetables. Small kohlrabi orbs don't need to be peeled; peel bigger orbs to decrease bitterness.

5. Heat ½ Tbs oil in a wok or frying pan, add the vegetables, and cook, stirring, 3-4 minutes or until just tender. If needed, add bone broth one Tbs at a time to keep from burning vegetables. Remove from pan.

6. Add the other ½ Tbs oil. Drain the marinade from the chicken and save it. Add the chicken to the hot oil and cook, stirring, about 2 minutes or until it turns white. If needed, add bone broth one Tbs at a time to keep from burning chicken.

7. Add vegetables and marinade and toss together 2 minutes, until the sauce thickens and the vegetables are hot.

Serves 2

Stovetop Fish

INGREDIENTS:

1 lb fish

2 medium leeks, white parts only

4 cloves garlic

1 Tbs coconut oil

1 tsp dried basil

1 tsp dried oregano

½ - 1 cup bone broth

Juice of one lemon

1 Tbs fresh tarragon, chopped

Sea salt and white pepper to taste

DIRECTIONS:

1. Cut off green tops of leeks and remove tough outer leaves. Cut off root end of leeks. Cut in half lengthwise. Fan out and rinse well but keep whole. Cut into 2-inch lengths and then cut into thin strips or ribbons.

2. Press garlic and allow leeks and garlic to sit for 5-10 minutes.

3. Cut fish into four servings. Rub fish with 1 Tbs lemon juice, salt, and pepper.

4. Heat oil in large skillet over medium heat. Add leeks, basil, and oregano. Sauté for about 5 minutes, stirring frequently.

5. Add garlic and sauté for an additional minute.

6. Add ½ cup broth and remaining lemon juice. Cover and simmer for 5 minutes, stirring occasionally. Add additional broth as necessary to keep from burning.

7. Stir in tarragon. Place fish on top of leeks. Simmer for 3-5 minutes, covered until fish flakes easily with fork.

Serves 4

Cooked Side Dishes

Artichokes

INGREDIENTS:

2 artichokes

1 tsp sea salt

2 garlic cloves, crushed

wedge of lemon

bay leaf

DIRECTIONS:

1. Crush garlic and allow to sit for 5-10 minutes.

2. Fill a pot about 1/3 full with water. Add salt, the garlic cloves, lemon wedge, and the bay leaf. Bring the water to a boil.

3. While the water is heating, wash the artichokes and cut off the tops (1/2" to 1" is usually sufficient). Cut off the stems flush with the bottoms so that the artichokes have flat bases. Peel off any bottom or exterior leaves that are too thick or tough. You can use scissors to trim off the prickly tips of the exterior leaves, if desired.

4. Place the artichokes in a steamer basket, place in pot and cover. Steam for 40-60 minutes depending on size.

5. Remove the artichokes, place upright on a plate, and serve.

EATING TIP: To eat, peel off individual leaves or petals. Tightly grip the "prickly" end of the petal. Place in mouth and pull through teeth to remove soft, pulpy, delicious portion of the petal. Discard remaining petal. Continue until all petals are removed. With a knife or spoon, scrape out and discard the inedible fuzzy part (called the "choke") covering the artichoke heart. The remaining bottom of the artichoke is the heart. Cut into pieces and eat.

Serves 1-2

Asparagus

INGREDIENTS:

1 lb asparagus

DRESSING:

1 Tbs extra virgin olive oil

1 tsp lemon juice

Sea salt

Fresh ground black pepper

DIRECTIONS:

1. Clean and trim asparagus. Remove woody part at end of stalk. Cut into 2 inch pieces.

2. Fill pot ¾ full with lightly salted water and bring to a boil.

3. Cook asparagus for 4-5 minutes or just until tender.

4. Drain. Toss with dressing ingredients. Serve.

Serves 2-4

Beet Greens

INGREDIENTS:

2 bunches beet greens
2 garlic cloves
1 Tbs coconut oil
¼ tsp red pepper flakes
1 tsp lemon juice
Sea salt
Fresh ground black pepper

DIRECTIONS:

1. Mince garlic and allow to sit for 5-10 minutes.

2. Wash beet greens. Remove stems and chop.

3. Bring a large pot of lightly salted water to a boil.

4. Prepare a bowl of ice water.

5. Add the beet greens to boiling water and cook uncovered until tender, 1-2 minutes.

6. Remove and immediately immerse in ice water for several minutes until cold to stop the cooking process.

7. Place in salad spinner and remove excess water.

8. Heat oil in a large skillet over medium heat. Sauté garlic and red pepper flakes until fragrant, about 1 minute. Stir in the greens until oil and garlic is evenly distributed and greens are warmed.

9. Season with salt, pepper, and lemon juice.

Serves 2-4

Beets—Steamed

INGREDIENTS:

1 lb medium sized beets

DRESSING:

3 Tbs extra virgin olive oil

2 tsp lemon juice

1 medium clove garlic

1 Tbs balsamic vinegar

1 Tbs fresh basil, minced

salt and cracked black pepper to taste

DIRECTIONS:

1. Fill the bottom of the steamer with 2 inches of water.

2. Chop or press garlic and allow to sit for 5-10 minutes.

3. Wash beets, peel, and cut into 1 inch cubes.

4. Steam covered for 15 minutes. Cooking is complete when you can easily insert a fork.

5. Transfer to a bowl, toss with dressing ingredients while still hot.

QUICK TIP: You can mellow the flavor of the garlic by adding it to the steamer for the last 2 minutes. Remember to wear gloves and an apron when cutting beets. You don't need to whisk together the dressing ingredients, just toss everything together at the end and serve.

Serves 2-4

Blanched Vegetables

Lightly boiling vegetables and then putting in an ice bath is called blanching. This is an easy and tasty way to eat vegetables, especially for people with digestive distress from raw foods. The directions are the same for all vegetables; just choose which ones you want to eat. Mix and match or eat only one vegetable. The choice is limitless. Boil, place in an ice bath, drain, and toss with dressing; try variations to find options you like best.

VEGETABLE	BOILING TIME
Asparagus	2-3 minutes
Beets	10-15 minutes
Broccoli	3 minutes
Brussel sprouts	3-5 minutes
Cabbage (wedges)	3 minutes
Carrots	3 minutes
Cauliflower	3 minutes
Collard greens	2 minutes
Leafy greens	2 minutes
Leeks	30-40 seconds
Okra	3-5 minutes
Parsnips	3 minutes
Summer Squash	3 minutes
Turnips	3 minutes

Blanched Vegetable Dressing

INGREDIENTS:

3 Tbs extra virgin olive oil (or flaxseed oil or combination of the two)

2 Tbs lemon juice

1 Tbs coconut aminos or balsamic vinegar

Sea salt and cracked black pepper to taste

Blanched Vegetable Dressing Add-ins:

2 Tbs sunflower seeds

2 Tbs fresh cilantro, chopped

2 Tbs fresh rosemary, chopped

2 Tbs fresh oregano, chopped

2 Tbs fresh thyme, chopped

2 Tbs fresh basil, chopped

1 tsp. turmeric

1 tsp. paprika

Pinch red pepper flakes

DIRECTIONS:

1. Cut vegetables into 2 inch pieces.
2. Fill pot ¾ full with lightly salted water and bring to a boil.
3. Cook just until tender crisp.
4. Prepare bowl of ice water.
5. Drain. Immerse vegetables in ice bath. Drain.
6. Toss with dressing ingredients. Serve.

Chard

INGREDIENTS:

1 clove garlic

1 lb Swiss chard

1 tsp fresh lemon juice

3 Tbs extra virgin olive oil

¼ tsp turmeric

1 tsp coconut aminos (optional)

Sea salt

Fresh ground black pepper

DIRECTIONS:

1. Press garlic and let sit for 5-10 minutes.

2. Using a large pot, fill ¾ full with water. Heat to boiling.

3. Rinse chard. Cut off tough, bottom part of Swiss chard stems. Cut white and rainbow chard stems into ½" slices. If using only red chard, discard stems. Cut leaves into 1" slices.

4. Add the chopped leaves/stems to the boiling water. Cook for 3 minutes; begin timing as soon as you drop the chard into the boiling water.

5. Place in salad spinner and remove excess water.

6. Transfer to serving dish and toss with rest of ingredients while it is still hot.

7. Using a knife and fork, cut Swiss chard into small pieces for better flavor.

Serves 2

Collard Greens

INGREDIENTS:

1 clove garlic

1 onion

1 lb collard greens

2 tsp + 2 tsp fresh lemon juice

3 Tbs extra virgin olive oil

Pinch of cayenne

Pinch of paprika

1 tsp coconut aminos (optional)

Sea salt

Fresh ground black pepper to taste

DIRECTIONS:

1. Press garlic and chop onion. Allow to sit for 5-10 minutes.

2. Rinse collard greens. Cut off tough bottom part of collard green stems. Cut leaves into ½" slices. Cut stems into ¼" slices. Cut crosswise as well to make small pieces.

3. Sprinkle with 2 tsp lemon juice and allow to sit for 5-10 minutes.

4. Using a large pot or steamer put 2 inches of water in the bottom of the pot. Bring to a rapid boil.

5. Place onions and chopped leaves/stems in steamer basket and place in pot. Cover and steam for 5 minutes. Begin timing as soon as you drop the steamer basket into the boiling water.

6. Quickly remove steamer basket. Put collard greens and onions in a salad spinner and remove excess water.

7. Transfer to serving dish and toss with rest of ingredients while it is still hot.

Serves 2

Kale

INGREDIENTS:

1 lb kale

1 clove garlic

2 tsp balsamic vinegar or apple cider vinegar

3 Tbs extra virgin olive oil

Sea salt

Fresh ground black pepper

¼ tsp allspice, ground coriander, cinnamon, and pinch of cloves (optional)

Chopped almonds (optional)

DIRECTIONS:

1. Press garlic and let sit for 5-10 minutes.

2. Chop kale and allow to sit for 5 minutes. Cut leaves into ½ inch slices until reaching stems then cut into ¼ inch slices.

3. Using a large pot or steamer put 2 inches of water in the bottom of the pot. Bring to a rapid boil.

4. Place leaves/stems in steamer basket and place in pot. Cover and steam for 5 minutes. Begin timing as soon as you drop the steamer basket into the boiling water.

5. Quickly remove steamer basket. Put kale in a salad spinner and remove excess water.

6. Toss with remaining ingredients.

7. Using a knife and fork, cut kale into small pieces.

QUICK TIP: You can mellow the flavor of the garlic by adding it to the steamer for the last 2 minutes.

Serves 2

Kohlrabi

INGREDIENTS FOR LEAVES:

1 pound fresh kohlrabi

1 tsp lemon juice

1 clove garlic

1 Tbs extra virgin olive oil

Sea salt

Fresh cracked black pepper

½ tsp coconut aminos (optional)

½ tsp sesame seeds (optional)

DIRECTIONS FOR LEAVES:

1. Press garlic and let it sit for 5-10 minutes.

2. Bring lightly salted water to a rapid boil in a large pot.

3. Cut stems and leaves off orbs and clean well.

4. Cook leaves in boiling water for 1 minute.

5. Drain and press out excess water. Toss in rest of ingredients while still hot.

INGREDIENTS FOR ORBS:

1 pound fresh kohlrabi

Sea salt

DIRECTIONS FOR ORBS:

1. Chop kohlrabi in 1-inch cubes.

2. Use a large pot (3 quart) and put 2 inches of water in the bottom of the pot. Make sure water is at a rapid boil.

3. Add kohlrabi to a steamer and place in pot. Cover. Steam for 5 minutes. Begin timing as soon as you drop the steamer basket into the boiling water.

4. Remove and sprinkle lightly with sea salt.

Steamed Vegetables

Steamed vegetables are easy and tasty. The directions are the same for all vegetables, just choose which ones you want to eat. Mix and match or eat only one vegetable. The choice is limitless. Steam and toss with dressing; try variations to find options you like best.

VEGETABLE	STEAM TIME:
Artichokes	40-60 minutes (see recipe)
Asparagus	2-4 minutes
Beets	15 minutes
Broccoli stems	5-7 minutes
Broccoli florets	4-5 minutes
Brussel sprouts	5-7 minutes
Cabbage	5-6 minutes
Carrots	5-7 minutes
Cauliflower	5-6 minutes
Celery	2 minutes
Collard greens	5 minutes
Kale	3-4 minutes
Mushrooms	3 minutes
Onion	3 minutes
Parsnips	7-8 minutes
Red onion	2 minutes
Summer Squash	3 minutes
Turnips	8-10 minutes
Winter Squash	7 minutes
Zucchini	3 minutes

Steamed Vegetable Dressing

INGREDIENTS:

3 Tbs extra virgin olive oil

2 Tbs lemon juice

2 medium cloves garlic

Sea salt and cracked black pepper to taste

Steamed Vegetable Dressing Add-ins:

½ tsp. coconut aminos

2 Tbs sunflower seeds

2 Tbs fresh cilantro, chopped

2 Tbs fresh rosemary, chopped

2 Tbs fresh oregano, chopped

2 Tbs fresh thyme, chopped

2 Tbs fresh basil, chopped

1 tsp. turmeric

1 tsp. paprika

Pinch red pepper flakes

DIRECTIONS:

1. Fill the bottom of the steamer with 2 inches of water.

2. Press garlic and allow to sit for 5-10 minutes.

3. Chop or slice vegetable into ¼ inch sections or 1 inch cubes. Allow to sit for 5-10 minutes.

4. Place vegetables in steamer basket. Add to pot. Cover and steam for designated time. Begin timing as soon as you drop the steamer basket into the boiling water.

5. Transfer to a bowl, toss with dressing ingredients while still hot.

QUICK TIP: You can mellow the flavor of the garlic by adding it to the steamer for the last 2 minutes. You don't need to whisk together the dressing ingredients, just toss everything together at the end and serve.

Spinach

INGREDIENTS:

1 pound fresh spinach

1 tsp apple cider vinegar

1 clove garlic, pressed or chopped

1 Tbs extra virgin olive oil

½ tsp coconut aminos (optional)

Sea salt

Fresh cracked black pepper

DIRECTIONS:

1. Press garlic and let it sit for 5-10 minutes.

2. Bring lightly salted water to a rapid boil in a large pot.

3. Cut stems off spinach leaves and clean well. This can be done easily by leaving spinach bundled and cutting off stems all at once. Rinse spinach leaves very well as they often contain a lot of soil.

4. Cook spinach in boiling water for 1 minute. Begin cooking time as soon as spinach is placed in water.

5. Place spinach in salad spinner and remove excess water.

6. Toss with remaining ingredients while still hot.

Serves 2

Spinach with Cranberries and Nuts

INGREDIENTS:

2 cloves garlic

½ small red onion

1 pound spinach leaves

2 Tbs coarsely chopped walnuts

1 Tbs coconut oil

½ cup cranberries

DIRECTIONS:

1. Thinly slice garlic and onion. Allow to sit for 5-10 minutes.

2. Sauté red onions in coconut oil over medium low heat for 5-10 minutes.

3. Turn up heat and add garlic to the pan, sauté lightly for an additional minute.

4. Bring lightly salted water to a rapid boil in a large pot.

5. Cut stems off spinach leaves and clean well. This can be done easily by leaving spinach bundled and cutting off stems all at once. Rinse spinach leaves very well as they often contain a lot of soil.

6. Cook spinach in boiling water for 1 minute. Begin cooking time as soon as spinach is placed in water.

7. Place spinach in salad spinner and remove excess water.

8. Toss all ingredients together. Serve.

Serves 2

Stuffed Mushrooms

INGREDIENTS:

1-2 cloves garlic

¼ cup shredded, unsweetened coconut

2 Portobello mushrooms

¼ cup finely chopped spinach

¼ cup macadamia nut oil

2 Tbs fresh lemon juice

½ tsp fresh grated lemon zest

½ tsp fresh grated ginger

2 Tbs sunflower seeds, ground

Sea salt

Fresh ground white pepper

1 Tbs fresh cilantro, chopped

DIRECTIONS:

1. Press garlic and let sit for 5-10 minutes.

2. Preheat oven to 400 degrees. Spread coconut on baking sheet and bake until slightly brown and fragrant.

3. Remove stems from mushrooms.

4. Combine coconut with remaining ingredients in a large bowl. Spoon the mixture into the mushrooms evenly. Cover loosely with foil and bake 15-20 minutes or until mushrooms are tender.

5. Broil for an additional minute to brown top.

6. Sprinkle with cilantro and serve.

Serves 1-2

Wilted Spinach Salad

INGREDIENTS:

6 cups baby spinach

DRESSING:

1 clove garlic

1 tsp apple cider vinegar

1 Tbs macadamia nut oil

1 oz. anchovies from jar

Sea salt

Fresh cracked black pepper

DIRECTIONS:

1. Press garlic and let it sit for 5-10 minutes.

2. Mix dressing ingredients in a small blender.

3. Warm dressing on stove, just a slight amount.

4. Drizzle dressing over baby spinach.

COOKING TIP: Be careful not to add too much dressing or it will cause the spinach to become overly wilted.

Serves 2

Raw Side Dishes

Beets—Basic Salad

INGREDIENTS:

3 medium beets

DRESSING:

3 Tbs flaxseed oil

1 Tbs fresh lemon juice

1 Tbs Dijon mustard

sea salt and pepper to taste

DIRECTIONS:

1. Peel and grate or shred beets.

2. Whisk together dressing. Season to taste.

3. Toss beets and dressing. Add to fresh greens of choice.

QUICK TIP: Remember to wear gloves and an apron when working with beets as they stain the skin and clothes. A food processor is quick and easy for shredding beets.

Serves 2

Beets—Raw Salad with Herbs

INGREDIENTS:

3 medium beets

DRESSING:

3 Tbs extra virgin olive oil

1 Tbs fresh lemon juice

2 Tbs mixed fresh herbs (basil, oregano and/or rosemary)

1 Tbs Dijon mustard (optional)

sea salt and pepper to taste

DIRECTIONS:

1. Peel and grate or shred beets.

2. Whisk together dressing. Season to taste.

3. Toss beets and dressing. Add to fresh greens of choice.

QUICK TIP: Remember to wear gloves and an apron when working with beets as they stain the skin and clothes. A food processor is quick and easy for shredding beets.

Serves 2

Cabbage

INGREDIENTS:

2 cups purple cabbage, shredded

½ cup radishes, thinly sliced

⅛ tsp cayenne pepper

1 Tbs coconut aminos

1 Tbs fresh lemon juice

½ Tbs organic lemon zest from peel

¼ tsp sea salt

1 green onion, minced

DIRECTIONS:

1. Combine all ingredients, except green onion. Mix well.

2. Marinate for 30 minutes.

3. Top with green onion.

QUICK TIP: Remember to wash lemon well before zesting or grating. Afterward, juice the lemon.

MAKE AHEAD ALERT: This recipe has to marinate. You can make ahead and allow to marinate for up to 2 days.

Serves 2

Cider Coleslaw

INGREDIENTS:

1 ½ cups shredded cabbage (red or green or combination)

1 carrot

1 apple, cored and chopped

1 cup apple cider vinegar

1 Tbs arrowroot powder

¼ tsp stevia (optional)

4 Tbs extra virgin olive oil

Sea salt to taste

3 green onions, diced

1 tsp caraway seeds (or to taste)

DIRECTIONS:

1. Shred cabbage and carrots in a food processor.

2. In a large bowl, toss cabbage, carrot, and apple to combine.

3. Use about 3 Tbs of the cider to make a smooth paste with arrowroot powder.

4. In a sauce pan, heat the remaining cider to boiling, add stevia if using, stir in arrowroot paste, and cook until clear.

5. Cool a little. Add olive oil and sea salt. Pour over cabbage, carrot, and apple. Mix well.

6. Sprinkle green onions and caraway seeds on top.

Serves 2

Cucumber Salad

INGREDIENTS:

1 bunch watercress, stems removed

1 cucumber

DRESSING:

4 tsp lemon juice

3 tsp flaxseed oil

¼ tsp sea salt

Fresh ground pepper to taste

DIRECTIONS:

1. Chop watercress. Halve, remove seeds, and thinly slice cucumber. Toss vegetables together.

2. Whisk together dressing.

3. Combine all ingredients. Lightly toss.

4. Serve.

Serves 2

Dandelion Salad

INGREDIENTS:

½ medium sized onion

2 Tbs apple cider vinegar

1 cup hot water

3 cups young dandelion greens

2 Tbs fresh basil, chopped

1 Tbs fresh tarragon, chopped

DRESSING:

1-½ Tbs balsamic vinegar

¼ tsp sea salt

¼ tsp coarse cracked black pepper

Extra virgin olive oil to taste

DIRECTIONS:

1. Thinly slice onion and place in a small bowl. Allow to sit 5-10 minutes.

2. Combine vinegar and water, pour over onions and marinate while making rest of salad.

3. Whisk together dressing ingredients adding oil at end a little at a time.

4. Rinse and chop dandelion greens. Dry greens.

5. Toss dandelion greens with ⅔ of the dressing.

6. Squeeze dry marinated onions and place on greens. Drizzle the rest of the dressing over salad. Top with herbs.

Serves 2

Kohlrabi

The flavor of this vegetable is delicately sweet and its texture is moist, yet crisp. It tastes mildly like broccoli with just a hint of cabbage.

DIRECTIONS:

1. Small orbs don't need to be peeled.
   Large orbs should be peeled to avoid bitterness.

2. Chop the leaves and add to lettuce or other greens.

3. Chop the orb and eat.

Marinated Cabbage Salad

INGREDIENTS:

½ head green cabbage

1 carrot

2 Tbs rice vinegar

3 Tbs extra virgin olive oil

½ cup chopped cilantro

1 Tbs chopped almonds

Sea salt to taste

DIRECTIONS:

1. Shred cabbage and carrot in a food processor.

2. Mix with remaining ingredients, except almonds.

3. Let marinate for ½ hour in refrigerator.

4. Toss with almonds and serve.

MAKE AHEAD ALERT: This recipe has to marinate. You can make ahead and allow to marinate for up to 2 days.

Serves 1

Quick Salad

INGREDIENTS:

¼ wedge red cabbage, shredded

1 carrot, chopped or shredded

1 beet, grated

4 stalks red chard, chopped

big handful arugula, chopped

½ cup organic broccoli sprouts

DRESSING:

3 Tbs extra virgin olive oil

1 Tbs fresh lemon juice

2 Tbs fresh tarragon

2 Tbs fresh rosemary

sea salt and pepper to taste

DIRECTIONS:

1. Shred cabbage, carrot, and beet in a food processor.

2. Whisk together dressing.

3. Combine all ingredients. Mix well.

QUICK TIP: Remember to wear gloves and an apron when working with beets as they stain the skin and clothes. A food processor is quick and easy for shredding beets.

Serves 1

Watercress Salad

INGREDIENTS:

1 bunch watercress

¾ cup butter lettuce

½ cucumber

5 radishes

½ carrot

DRESSING:

3 Tbs flaxseed oil

1 Tbs lemon juice

½ cup filtered water

3 Tbs rice vinegar

3 Tbs coconut aminos

2 Tbs mirin

DIRECTIONS:

1. Chop watercress and lettuce. Halve, remove seeds, and thinly slice cucumber. Thinly slice radishes. Shred carrot. Toss vegetables together.

2. Whisk together dressing.

3. Combine all ingredients. Lightly toss. Marinate for 30 minutes.

4. Serve.

MAKE AHEAD ALERT: This recipe has to marinate for 30 minutes.

Serves 2

Zucchini Salad

INGREDIENTS:

1 pounds zucchini

3 Tbs flaxseed oil

1 Tbs fresh lemon juice

½ tsp sea salt

¼ tsp fresh ground black pepper

pinch dried red pepper flakes

¼ cup chopped fresh basil

2 Tbs pine nuts

DIRECTIONS:

1. Place pine nuts in shallow skillet and toast until golden brown and fragrant.

2. Whisk oil, lemon juice, salt, and peppers in a small bowl. Set dressing aside.

3. Using a slicer or mandolin, work from the top to bottom of each zucchini, slicing into ribbons about $\frac{1}{16}$ inch thick. Place in a large bowl.

4. Add basil and nuts to zucchini ribbons.

5. Add dressing to zucchini ribbons. Toss to coat.

6. Season with additional salt and pepper to taste.

HELPFUL HINT: Skip toasting the pine nuts if you are in a hurry.

Serves 2

Dinners

Almond Onion Soup

INGREDIENTS:

2 cups raw almonds

4 cups warm filtered water

2 Tbs fresh lemon juice

2 onions

2 Tbs coconut oil

3 cups bone broth

2 tsp dried marjoram

2 tsp dried thyme

Sea salt

Fresh ground white pepper

DIRECTIONS:

1. Place almonds in bowl with water and lemon juice. Allow to soak overnight.

2. Drain almonds.

3. Chop onions and allow to sit for 5-10 minutes.

4. In a soup pot heat coconut oil and sauté onions over medium heat for 5 minutes.

5. Add all remaining ingredients. Using an immersion blender, blend until smooth. You can also process in a food processor or blender in batches.

6. Warm to desired temperature. Add additional seasonings as desired.

Serves 3

Borscht Soup

INGREDIENTS:

1 beet, peeled and cut into chunks

1 cucumber, peeled and cut into chunks

1 avocado, cubed

2 green onions, chopped

1 lemon, juiced

Small handful of dill

Extra virgin olive oil

Sea salt

Fresh ground pepper

DIRECTIONS:

1. Combine all ingredients in a blender. Blend until smooth.

2. Add water if needed to thin soup.

3. Adjust seasonings to taste.

4. Warm slightly, if desired.

Serves 1

Coconut Thai Soup

INGREDIENTS:

2 ½ cups bone broth

1 can BPA-free coconut milk

2 Tbs fresh lemon juice

2 Tbs tamari

¼ cup fresh grated ginger

zest and juice of one lime

1 Tbs chili paste

DIRECTIONS:

1. Place all ingredients in a large saucepan. Using an immersion blender, blend until smooth. You can also process in a food processor or blender in batches.

2. Warm to desired level.

Serves 2

Creamy Carrot Soup

INGREDIENTS:

1 pound carrots

3 cloves garlic

1 medium onion

1 Tbs coconut oil

1 cup bone broth

½ cup BPA-free canned coconut milk

¼ cup hazelnut milk

1 tsp. fresh ginger, grated

Sea salt

Fresh ground white pepper

1 Tbs parsley, finely chopped

DIRECTIONS:

1. Fill the bottom of a steamer with 2 inches of water.

2. Chop garlic and onion. Allow to sit for 5-10 minutes.

3. Chop carrots into ½ inch sections or 1 inch cubes.

4. Once water is boiling, add carrots to steamer basket. Cover and steam for 5 minutes.

5. In a soup pot heat coconut oil and sauté onions over medium heat for 5 minutes.

6. Add garlic and sauté an additional minute.

7. Add carrots to pot. Using an immersion blender, blend until smooth. You can also process in a food processor or blender in batches.

8. Add remaining ingredients except parsley. Heat to desired temperature.

9. After placing in serving bowl, sprinkle parsley on top.

Serves 3

Mushroom Soup

INGREDIENTS:

1 medium onion

3 cloves garlic

2 stalks celery

2 carrots

1 Tbs coconut oil

1 cup sliced shiitake mushrooms

1 cup sliced crimini mushrooms

½ Tbs dried rosemary

½ Tbs dried sage

½ Tbs dried thyme

3 cups bone broth

2 Tbs miso paste

2 bay leaves

1 tsp turmeric

Sea salt

Fresh ground pepper

DIRECTIONS:

1. Chop onion and press garlic. Allow to sit for 5-10 minutes.

2. Chop celery and carrots.

3. In a soup pot heat coconut oil and sauté onions, celery, rosemary, sage, and thyme over medium heat for 5 minutes.

4. Add garlic and sauté an additional minute.

5. Add carrots and mushrooms and sauté for another 3 minutes. Add bone broth to prevent burning.

6. Add broth, miso, bay leaves, and turmeric. Bring to a light boil, reduce heat and simmer for 20-30 minutes.

7. Remove bay leaves. Add seasonings to desired taste.

Serves 3

Pozole Soup

INGREDIENTS:

1 medium onion

3 medium cloves garlic

½ poblano pepper, diced

1 Tbs coconut oil

4 cups bone broth

2 Tbs fresh lime juice

5-10 whole peppercorns

1 Tbs dried oregano

4 large tomatoes, chopped or 15 oz can diced tomatoes

3 carrots, sliced or grated

1 red pepper, chopped

3 stocks celery, chopped

1 fennel bulb, chopped

2 cups butternut squash, cubed

½ tsp cumin

1 tsp chili powder

3 cups kale, chopped

3-4 Tbs fresh cilantro, chopped

sea salt and pepper to taste

DIRECTIONS:

1. Chop onion and mince garlic. Allow to sit for 5-10 minutes.

2. Dice poblano pepper. Rinse kale and remove stems. Chop fine.

3. Sauté onion and pepper in coconut oil 3-5 minutes. Add garlic and sauté for another minute.

4. Add broth, lime juice, peppercorns, and oregano. Bring to a boil on high heat.

5. Add tomatoes, carrots, red pepper, celery, fennel, squash, cumin, and chili powder. Reduce heat to medium low and simmer for 20 minutes uncovered.

6. Add kale. Cook for 5 more minutes.

7. Add cilantro, salt, and pepper. Best if allowed to cool and served the following day.

Serves 4

Red Pepper Artichoke Soup

INGREDIENTS:

Head of garlic

4 red peppers or 15 oz jar of roasted red peppers

2 Tbs coconut oil

½ cup chopped onions

1 ½ cups bone broth

½ cup BPA-free canned coconut milk

½ cup almond milk

1 Tbs coconut oil

2 cups cooked artichokes or 15 oz jar artichokes

¼ cup chopped parsley leaves

Sea salt

White pepper

Pinch of cayenne (optional)

Smoked paprika (optional)

Macadamia nut oil

DIRECTIONS:

1. To roast red peppers: Preheat broiler. Melt coconut oil. Quarter and seed peppers. Brush peppers with coconut oil. Place under broiler until skins are thoroughly blistered and blackened. Allow to cool. Peel peppers discarding skins.

2. To roast garlic head: Remove outer skin of head of garlic. Cut the top off between ⅛-¼ inch down. Spread a bit of coconut oil over the top and wrap in foil. Put in oven with red peppers or roast separately. Using a pot holder carefully squeeze the head; it is done when it's very soft. Usually about 30 minutes in a 400 degree oven.

3. Chop onions and allow to sit 5-10 minutes.

4. Sauté onions in coconut oil.

5. Drain artichokes if using jarred. Drain red peppers if using jarred.

6. Place broth, milks, onions, garlic, and ½ of the artichokes in a food processor or blender. Blend until smooth. Add to pot used for sautéing onions.

7. Place remaining artichokes, peppers, and parsley in food processor and pulse until these items are chopped well, or chop by hand. Add to pot.

8. Season with spices to desired taste and warm to desired level.

9. After placing in serving bowl, drizzle oil on top.

HELPFUL TIP: In a hurry? Just mince the garlic and throw it in. The soup has a richer flavor with roasted garlic but time may be of the essence.

Serves 4

Spicy Soup

INGREDIENTS:

1 medium onion

4 garlic cloves

1 Tbs coconut oil

2 Tbs chili powder

3 cups bone broth

1 medium green pepper

1 poblano pepper

3 small tomatoes

1 tsp dried oregano

1 tsp ground cumin

1 small zucchini

4 collard green leaves

½ cup fresh cilantro

¼ cup pumpkin seeds

Sea salt

Fresh ground pepper

DIRECTIONS:

1. Mince onion and chop garlic. Allow to sit for 5-10 minutes.

2. Dice green pepper and zucchini into ¼ inch pieces.

3. Finely chop collard greens. Dice tomato and poblano.

4. Chop pumpkin seeds and cilantro.

5. Heat oil in a medium soup pot. Sauté onion, green peppers, and poblano over medium heat for about 5 minutes, stirring often.

6. Add garlic and sauté an additional minute.

7. Add red chili powder and mix in well. Add broth and tomatoes. Cook for another 5 minutes. Add oregano and cumin.

8. Bring to a boil on high heat. Once it begins to boil, reduce heat to medium-low and simmer uncovered for 10 minutes longer.

9. Add zucchini and collard greens and cook for 5 more minutes. Add chopped cilantro, pumpkin seeds, salt, and pepper.

Serves 6

Squash Soup

INGREDIENTS:

2 cups butternut squash, or any variety of winter squash, cut into 1-inch cubes

1 tsp lemon juice

1 ½ cups bone broth

3 Tbs BPA-free canned coconut milk

1 Tbs chopped fresh ginger

1 tsp turmeric

Sea Salt

Fresh ground white pepper

Macadamia nut oil

DIRECTIONS:

1. Fill the bottom of a steamer with 2 inches of water.

2. While steam is building up in steamer, peel and cut squash into 1-inch cubes.

3. Steam covered for 7 minutes. Squash is done when it is tender, yet still firm enough to hold its shape.

4. Place squash in pan and add remaining ingredients.

5. Heat to desired temperature.

6. Using an immersion blender, blend until smooth. You can also process in a food processor or blender in batches.

7. After placing in serving bowl, drizzle oil on top.

Serves 2

Vegetable Soup

INGREDIENTS:

2 carrots

2 celery stocks

½ onion

½ leek

1 cup cabbage

2 cups broccoli

1 garlic clove

4 cups bone broth

1 tsp curry powder

1 tsp fresh lemon juice

Sea salt

Fresh ground pepper

Toasted pine nuts or walnuts

DIRECTIONS:

1. Chop all vegetables in ½-1 inch pieces. Let them sit for 5 minutes.

2. Place vegetables in a pot. Add remaining ingredients, except nuts.

3. Bring to boiling over high heat. Reduce heat and simmer for 15-20 minutes until vegetables are cooked through.

4. Using an immersion blender, blend until smooth. You can also process in a food processor or blender in batches.

5. Add seasonings to preferred taste.

6. Top with desired nuts before serving.

Serves 2-4

Journal

My Food Journal: Day 1

Good luck on your journey to optimal health.

DATE: _____

Write down everything you eat and drink including all snacks, beverages, and water. If you notice any mood or digestive changes associated with a meal/snack, record it. Write a positive affirmation each day. Note the other cleansing technique used today as well as duration and type of exercise completed.

MEAL/ BEVERAGE	MOOD/ DIGESTIVE CHANGES	AFFIRMATION	CLEANSE/ EXERCISE
BREAKFAST *Time:*			
SNACK *Time:*			
LUNCH *Time:*			
SNACK *Time:*			
DINNER *Time:*			
SNACK *Time:*			

My Food Journal: Day 2

DATE: _____

Write down everything you eat and drink including all snacks, beverages, and water. If you notice any mood or digestive changes associated with a meal/snack, record it. Write a positive affirmation each day. Note the other cleansing technique used today as well as duration and type of exercise completed.

MEAL/ BEVERAGE	MOOD/ DIGESTIVE CHANGES	AFFIRMATION	CLEANSE/ EXERCISE
BREAKFAST *Time:*			
SNACK *Time:*			
LUNCH *Time:*			
SNACK *Time:*			
DINNER *Time:*			
SNACK *Time:*			

My Food Journal: Day 3

DATE: _____

Write down everything you eat and drink including all snacks, beverages, and water. If you notice any mood or digestive changes associated with a meal/snack, record it. Write a positive affirmation each day. Note the other cleansing technique used today as well as duration and type of exercise completed.

MEAL/ BEVERAGE	MOOD/ DIGESTIVE CHANGES	AFFIRMATION	CLEANSE/ EXERCISE
BREAKFAST *Time:*			
SNACK *Time:*			
LUNCH *Time:*			
SNACK *Time:*			
DINNER *Time:*			
SNACK *Time:*			

My Food Journal: Day 4

DATE: _____

Write down everything you eat and drink including all snacks, beverages, and water. If you notice any mood or digestive changes associated with a meal/snack, record it. Write a positive affirmation each day. Note the other cleansing technique used today as well as duration and type of exercise completed.

MEAL/ BEVERAGE	MOOD/ DIGESTIVE CHANGES	AFFIRMATION	CLEANSE/ EXERCISE
BREAKFAST *Time:*			
SNACK *Time:*			
LUNCH *Time:*			
SNACK *Time:*			
DINNER *Time:*			
SNACK *Time:*			

My Food Journal: Day 5

Preparation week is almost over.

DATE: _____

Write down everything you eat and drink including all snacks, beverages, and water. If you notice any mood or digestive changes associated with a meal/snack, record it. Write a positive affirmation each day. Note the other cleansing technique used today as well as duration and type of exercise completed.

MEAL/ BEVERAGE	MOOD/ DIGESTIVE CHANGES	AFFIRMATION	CLEANSE/ EXERCISE
BREAKFAST *Time:*			
SNACK *Time:*			
LUNCH *Time:*			
SNACK *Time:*			
DINNER *Time:*			
SNACK *Time:*			

My Food Journal: Day 6

DATE: _____

Write down everything you eat and drink including all snacks, beverages, and water. If you notice any mood or digestive changes associated with a meal/snack, record it. Write a positive affirmation each day. Note the other cleansing technique used today as well as duration and type of exercise completed.

MEAL/ BEVERAGE	MOOD/ DIGESTIVE CHANGES	AFFIRMATION	CLEANSE/ EXERCISE
BREAKFAST *Time:*			
SNACK *Time:*			
LUNCH *Time:*			
SNACK *Time:*			
DINNER *Time:*			
SNACK *Time:*			

My Food Journal: Day 7

Congrats you've made it through preparation.

DATE: _____

Write down everything you eat and drink including all snacks, beverages, and water. If you notice any mood or digestive changes associated with a meal/snack, record it. Write a positive affirmation each day. Note the other cleansing technique used today as well as duration and type of exercise completed.

MEAL/ BEVERAGE	MOOD/ DIGESTIVE CHANGES	AFFIRMATION	CLEANSE/ EXERCISE
BREAKFAST *Time:*			
SNACK *Time:*			
LUNCH *Time:*			
SNACK *Time:*			
DINNER *Time:*			
SNACK *Time:*			

My Food Journal: Day 8

DATE: _____

Write down everything you eat and drink including all snacks, beverages, and water. If you notice any mood or digestive changes associated with a meal/snack, record it. Write a positive affirmation each day. Note the other cleansing technique used today as well as duration and type of exercise completed.

MEAL/ BEVERAGE	MOOD/ DIGESTIVE CHANGES	AFFIRMATION	CLEANSE/ EXERCISE
BREAKFAST *Time:*			
SNACK *Time:*			
LUNCH *Time:*			
SNACK *Time:*			
DINNER *Time:*			
SNACK *Time:*			

My Food Journal: Day 9

DATE: _____

Write down everything you eat and drink including all snacks, beverages, and water. If you notice any mood or digestive changes associated with a meal/snack, record it. Write a positive affirmation each day. Note the other cleansing technique used today as well as duration and type of exercise completed.

MEAL/ BEVERAGE	MOOD/ DIGESTIVE CHANGES	AFFIRMATION	CLEANSE/ EXERCISE
BREAKFAST *Time:*			
SNACK *Time:*			
LUNCH *Time:*			
SNACK *Time:*			
DINNER *Time:*			
SNACK *Time:*			

My Food Journal: Day 10

DATE: _____

Write down everything you eat and drink including all snacks, beverages, and water. If you notice any mood or digestive changes associated with a meal/snack, record it. Write a positive affirmation each day. Note the other cleansing technique used today as well as duration and type of exercise completed.

MEAL/ BEVERAGE	MOOD/ DIGESTIVE CHANGES	AFFIRMATION	CLEANSE/ EXERCISE
BREAKFAST *Time:*			
SNACK *Time:*			
LUNCH *Time:*			
SNACK *Time:*			
DINNER *Time:*			
SNACK *Time:*			

My Food Journal: Day 11

Keep up the great work.

DATE: _____

Write down everything you eat and drink including all snacks, beverages, and water. If you notice any mood or digestive changes associated with a meal/snack, record it. Write a positive affirmation each day. Note the other cleansing technique used today as well as duration and type of exercise completed.

MEAL/ BEVERAGE	MOOD/ DIGESTIVE CHANGES	AFFIRMATION	CLEANSE/ EXERCISE
BREAKFAST *Time:*			
SNACK *Time:*			
LUNCH *Time:*			
SNACK *Time:*			
DINNER *Time:*			
SNACK *Time:*			

My Food Journal: Day 12

DATE: _____

Write down everything you eat and drink including all snacks, beverages, and water. If you notice any mood or digestive changes associated with a meal/snack, record it. Write a positive affirmation each day. Note the other cleansing technique used today as well as duration and type of exercise completed.

MEAL/ BEVERAGE	MOOD/ DIGESTIVE CHANGES	AFFIRMATION	CLEANSE/ EXERCISE
BREAKFAST *Time:*			
SNACK *Time:*			
LUNCH *Time:*			
SNACK *Time:*			
DINNER *Time:*			
SNACK *Time:*			

My Food Journal: Day 13

DATE: _____

Write down everything you eat and drink including all snacks, beverages, and water. If you notice any mood or digestive changes associated with a meal/snack, record it. Write a positive affirmation each day. Note the other cleansing technique used today as well as duration and type of exercise completed.

MEAL/ BEVERAGE	MOOD/ DIGESTIVE CHANGES	AFFIRMATION	CLEANSE/ EXERCISE
BREAKFAST *Time:*			
SNACK *Time:*			
LUNCH *Time:*			
SNACK *Time:*			
DINNER *Time:*			
SNACK *Time:*			

My Food Journal: Day 14

Congrats you made it through the first week.

DATE: _____

Write down everything you eat and drink including all snacks, beverages, and water. If you notice any mood or digestive changes associated with a meal/snack, record it. Write a positive affirmation each day. Note the other cleansing technique used today as well as duration and type of exercise completed.

MEAL/ BEVERAGE	MOOD/ DIGESTIVE CHANGES	AFFIRMATION	CLEANSE/ EXERCISE
BREAKFAST Time:			
SNACK Time:			
LUNCH Time:			
SNACK Time:			
DINNER Time:			
SNACK Time:			

My Food Journal: Day 15

DATE: _____

Write down everything you eat and drink including all snacks, beverages, and water. If you notice any mood or digestive changes associated with a meal/snack, record it. Write a positive affirmation each day. Note the other cleansing technique used today as well as duration and type of exercise completed.

MEAL/ BEVERAGE	MOOD/ DIGESTIVE CHANGES	AFFIRMATION	CLEANSE/ EXERCISE
BREAKFAST *Time:*			
SNACK *Time:*			
LUNCH *Time:*			
SNACK *Time:*			
DINNER *Time:*			
SNACK *Time:*			

My Food Journal: Day 16

DATE: _____

Write down everything you eat and drink including all snacks, beverages, and water. If you notice any mood or digestive changes associated with a meal/snack, record it. Write a positive affirmation each day. Note the other cleansing technique used today as well as duration and type of exercise completed.

MEAL/ BEVERAGE	MOOD/ DIGESTIVE CHANGES	AFFIRMATION	CLEANSE/ EXERCISE
BREAKFAST *Time:*			
SNACK *Time:*			
LUNCH *Time:*			
SNACK *Time:*			
DINNER *Time:*			
SNACK *Time:*			

My Food Journal: Day 17

DATE: _____

Write down everything you eat and drink including all snacks, beverages, and water. If you notice any mood or digestive changes associated with a meal/snack, record it. Write a positive affirmation each day. Note the other cleansing technique used today as well as duration and type of exercise completed.

MEAL/ BEVERAGE	MOOD/ DIGESTIVE CHANGES	AFFIRMATION	CLEANSE/ EXERCISE
BREAKFAST *Time:*			
SNACK *Time:*			
LUNCH *Time:*			
SNACK *Time:*			
DINNER *Time:*			
SNACK *Time:*			

My Food Journal: Day 18

DATE: _____

Write down everything you eat and drink including all snacks, beverages, and water. If you notice any mood or digestive changes associated with a meal/snack, record it. Write a positive affirmation each day. Note the other cleansing technique used today as well as duration and type of exercise completed.

MEAL/ BEVERAGE	MOOD/ DIGESTIVE CHANGES	AFFIRMATION	CLEANSE/ EXERCISE
BREAKFAST *Time:*			
SNACK *Time:*			
LUNCH *Time:*			
SNACK *Time:*			
DINNER *Time:*			
SNACK *Time:*			

My Food Journal: Day 19

DATE: _____

Write down everything you eat and drink including all snacks, beverages, and water. If you notice any mood or digestive changes associated with a meal/snack, record it. Write a positive affirmation each day. Note the other cleansing technique used today as well as duration and type of exercise completed.

MEAL/ BEVERAGE	MOOD/ DIGESTIVE CHANGES	AFFIRMATION	CLEANSE/ EXERCISE
BREAKFAST *Time:*			
SNACK *Time:*			
LUNCH *Time:*			
SNACK *Time:*			
DINNER *Time:*			
SNACK *Time:*			

My Food Journal: Day 20

DATE: _____

Write down everything you eat and drink including all snacks, beverages, and water. If you notice any mood or digestive changes associated with a meal/snack, record it. Write a positive affirmation each day. Note the other cleansing technique used today as well as duration and type of exercise completed.

MEAL/ BEVERAGE	MOOD/ DIGESTIVE CHANGES	AFFIRMATION	CLEANSE/ EXERCISE
BREAKFAST *Time:*			
SNACK *Time:*			
LUNCH *Time:*			
SNACK *Time:*			
DINNER *Time:*			
SNACK *Time:*			

My Food Journal: Day 21

DATE: _____

Write down everything you eat and drink including all snacks, beverages, and water. If you notice any mood or digestive changes associated with a meal/snack, record it. Write a positive affirmation each day. Note the other cleansing technique used today as well as duration and type of exercise completed.

MEAL/ BEVERAGE	MOOD/ DIGESTIVE CHANGES	AFFIRMATION	CLEANSE/ EXERCISE
BREAKFAST *Time:*			
SNACK *Time:*			
LUNCH *Time:*			
SNACK *Time:*			
DINNER *Time:*			
SNACK *Time:*			

My Food Journal: Day 22

DATE: _____

Write down everything you eat and drink including all snacks, beverages, and water. If you notice any mood or digestive changes associated with a meal/snack, record it. Write a positive affirmation each day. Note the other cleansing technique used today as well as duration and type of exercise completed.

MEAL/ BEVERAGE	MOOD/ DIGESTIVE CHANGES	AFFIRMATION	CLEANSE/ EXERCISE
BREAKFAST *Time:*			
SNACK *Time:*			
LUNCH *Time:*			
SNACK *Time:*			
DINNER *Time:*			
SNACK *Time:*			

My Food Journal: Day 23

DATE: _____

Write down everything you eat and drink including all snacks, beverages, and water. If you notice any mood or digestive changes associated with a meal/snack, record it. Write a positive affirmation each day. Note the other cleansing technique used today as well as duration and type of exercise completed.

MEAL/ BEVERAGE	MOOD/ DIGESTIVE CHANGES	AFFIRMATION	CLEANSE/ EXERCISE
BREAKFAST *Time:*			
SNACK *Time:*			
LUNCH *Time:*			
SNACK *Time:*			
DINNER *Time:*			
SNACK *Time:*			

My Food Journal: Day 24

DATE: _____

Write down everything you eat and drink including all snacks, beverages, and water. If you notice any mood or digestive changes associated with a meal/snack, record it. Write a positive affirmation each day. Note the other cleansing technique used today as well as duration and type of exercise completed.

MEAL/ BEVERAGE	MOOD/ DIGESTIVE CHANGES	AFFIRMATION	CLEANSE/ EXERCISE
BREAKFAST *Time:*			
SNACK *Time:*			
LUNCH *Time:*			
SNACK *Time:*			
DINNER *Time:*			
SNACK *Time:*			

My Food Journal: Day 25

Only a few days left.

DATE: _____

Write down everything you eat and drink including all snacks, beverages, and water. If you notice any mood or digestive changes associated with a meal/snack, record it. Write a positive affirmation each day. Note the other cleansing technique used today as well as duration and type of exercise completed.

MEAL/ BEVERAGE	MOOD/ DIGESTIVE CHANGES	AFFIRMATION	CLEANSE/ EXERCISE
BREAKFAST *Time:*			
SNACK *Time:*			
LUNCH *Time:*			
SNACK *Time:*			
DINNER *Time:*			
SNACK *Time:*			

My Food Journal: Day 26

DATE: _____

Write down everything you eat and drink including all snacks, beverages, and water. If you notice any mood or digestive changes associated with a meal/snack, record it. Write a positive affirmation each day. Note the other cleansing technique used today as well as duration and type of exercise completed.

MEAL/ BEVERAGE	MOOD/ DIGESTIVE CHANGES	AFFIRMATION	CLEANSE/ EXERCISE
BREAKFAST Time:			
SNACK Time:			
LUNCH Time:			
SNACK Time:			
DINNER Time:			
SNACK Time:			

My Food Journal: Day 27

DATE: _____

Write down everything you eat and drink including all snacks, beverages, and water. If you notice any mood or digestive changes associated with a meal/snack, record it. Write a positive affirmation each day. Note the other cleansing technique used today as well as duration and type of exercise completed.

MEAL/ BEVERAGE	MOOD/ DIGESTIVE CHANGES	AFFIRMATION	CLEANSE/ EXERCISE
BREAKFAST *Time:*			
SNACK *Time:*			
LUNCH *Time:*			
SNACK *Time:*			
DINNER *Time:*			
SNACK *Time:*			

My Food Journal: Day 28

Congrats! You've completed the journey.

DATE: _____

Write down everything you eat and drink including all snacks, beverages, and water. If you notice any mood or digestive changes associated with a meal/snack, record it. Write a positive affirmation each day. Note the other cleansing technique used today as well as duration and type of exercise completed.

MEAL/ BEVERAGE	MOOD/ DIGESTIVE CHANGES	AFFIRMATION	CLEANSE/ EXERCISE
BREAKFAST *Time:*			
SNACK *Time:*			
LUNCH *Time:*			
SNACK *Time:*			
DINNER *Time:*			
SNACK *Time:*			

Sources and Recommended Reading

Barringer, Caroline. (2010). Immunitrition.
http://www.immunitrition.com.

Batmanghelidj, F. MD. (2008). *Your Body's Many Cries for Water*. Decatur, GA: Global Health Solutions, Inc.

Bralley, J. Alexander and Richard S. Lord. (1999). *Amino Acids in Laboratory Evaluations in Nutritional Medicine*. Norcross, GA: MetaMetrix.

Brody, Tom. (1999). *Nutritional Biochemistry*. San Diego, CA: Academic Press.

Campbell-McBride, Natasha Dr. (2010). *Gut and Psychology Syndrome*. Soham, Cambridge: Medinform Publishing.

Center For Food Safety. (2012). http://truefoodnow.org/campaigns/ genetically-engineered-foods.

Daniel, Kaayla. (2003). Why Broth is Beautiful: Essential Roles for Proline, Glycine and Gelatin. *Wise Traditions in Food, Farming and the Healing Arts*. Vol.4, 1.

Espinoza, Jessica. (2011). Delicious Obsessions.
http://www.deliciousobsessions.com.

Fallon, Sally. (2000). *Broth is Beautiful*. Retrieved June 7, 2010 from http://www.westonaprice.org.

Fallon, Sally & Mary Enig. (2001). *Nourishing Traditions: The Cookbook that Challenges Politically Correct Nutrition and the Diet Dictocrats*. Washington, DC: NewTrends Publishing, Inc.

Floyd, Margaret. (2011). *Eat Naked: Unprocessed, Unpolluted, and Undressed Eating for a Healthier, Sexier You*. Oakland, CA: New Harbinger Publications, Inc.

Haas, Elson M. MD. (2006). *Staying Healthy with Nutrition*. Berkely, CA: Celestial Arts.

Huber, Colleen Dr. (2007). *Choose Your Foods Like Your Life Depends on Them*. Bloomington, IN: Xlibris Corporation.

Lubec, G, et al. (1989). Amino acid isomerisation and microwave *exposure*. Lancet. Vol. 2, 8676: 1392-1393.

Mateljan, George. (2007). *The World's Healthiest Foods*. Seattle, WA: George Mateljan Foundation.

McGruther, Jenny. (2011). Nourished Kitchen.
http://www.nourishedkitchen.com.

Ottenberg, Reuben Dr. (1935). Painless Jaundice. *Journal of the American Medical Association, Vol. 104, 9: 1681-1687*

Pitchford, Paul. (2002). *Healing with Whole Foods.* Berkeley, CA: North Atlantic Books.

Pope, Sarah. (2012). *The Bountiful Benefits of Bone Broths.* Presented July, 2012 at Real Food Summit. http://realfoodsummit.com/sarah-pope.

Pope, Sarah. (2010). The Healthy Home Economist. http://www.thehealthyhomeeconomist.com.

Resnick, Donald & Niwayama, Gen. (1988). *Diagnosis of Bone and Joint Disorders.* Philadelphia: WB Saunders

Richardson, CT, et al. (1976). Studies on the mechanism of food-stimulated gastric acid secretion in normal human subjects. *Journal of Clinical Investigation. Vol. 58: 623-631.*

Ross, Patricia Dr. & Scott Sharp Armstrong. (2007). *The Best Affirmations Workbook.* Self published. http://www.bestaffirmationscoach.com.

Shacter, Emily. (2002). Quantification and Significance of Protein Oxidation in Biological Samples. *Drug Metabolism Reviews. Vol. 32: 307-326.*

Shanahan, Dr. Catherine & Luke Shanahan. (2009). *Deep Nutrition. Big Box Books:* Lawai HI.

Singh A, Purohit B. (2011). Tooth brushing, oil pulling and tissue regeneration: A review of holistic approaches to oral health. *J Ayurveda Integr Med. Vol 2:64-68.*

Sizer, Frances & Whitney, Ellie (2008). *Nutrition: The Science of Eating.* Mason, OH: Cengage Learning.

Stanfield, Peggy & Y.H. Hui. (2003). *Nutrition and Diet Therapy.* Sudbury, MA: Jones and Barlett Publishers.

Thibodeau, Gary A. & Patton, Kevin T. (2008). *Structure and Function of the Body.* St. Louis, MI: Mosby Elsevier.

Weston A. Price Foundation. (2009). For Wise Traditions in Food, Farming, and the Healing Arts. http://www.westonaprice.org.

Recipe Index

About the Author

After receiving a Bachelor of Arts degree in Speech Communication, Kellie started her career in the world of non-profit. The opportunity to "learn business the old-fashioned way" led her to purchase the first of two 7-Eleven franchises. After five years, and meeting her soon-to-be-husband, she sold her businesses and took the opportunity to learn the McDonald's restaurant business. She worked her way up through the system and became an approved owner/operator. After ten years in the fast food industry she realized her continuous passion for nutrition was her true calling.

Kellie went back to school receiving a Bachelor of Science in Nutrition, Health and Wellness. Wanting to find even healthier alternatives to offer clients, she received her Nutritional Therapy Practitioner certification the following year.

Years of working with private clients and instructing cooking classes led Kellie to want to produce programs for individuals that didn't have the desire or resources to be a private client. The Cleanse and Detoxify Your Body Program is one of the results.

Contact

You can contact Kellie through her website at therightnutritionplan.com, email to kellie@therightnutritionplan.com,
snail mail to The Right Plan 706 Cardley Avenue Medford OR 97504,
phone 541-772-PLAN (7526) or 1-855-772-PLAN (7526),
Facebook at www.facebook.com/TheRightPlan,
and Twitter at twitter.com/TheRightPlan.

Made in the USA
San Bernardino, CA
25 January 2015